Medical Education in Psychiatry

Editors

ROBERT J. BOLAND
HERMIONI L. AMONOO

PSYCHIATRIC CLINICS
OF NORTH AMERICA

www.psych.theclinics.com

Consulting Editor
HARSH K. TRIVEDI

June 2021 • Volume 44 • Number 2

ELSEVIER

1600 John F. Kennedy Boulevard • Suite 1800 • Philadelphia, Pennsylvania, 19103-2899

http://www.theclinics.com

PSYCHIATRIC CLINICS OF NORTH AMERICA Volume 44, Number 2
June 2021 ISSN 0193-953X, ISBN-13: 978-0-323-77831-2

Editor: Lauren Boyle
Developmental Editor: Diana Ang

Psychiatric Clinics of North America (ISSN 0193-953X) is published quarterly by Elsevier Inc., 360 Park Avenue South, New York, NY 10010-1710. Months of issue are March, June, September, and December. Business and Editorial Offices: 1600 John F. Kennedy Blvd., Suite 1800, Philadelphia, PA 19103-2899. Periodicals postage paid at New York, NY and additional mailing offices. Subscription prices are $338.00 per year (US individuals), $966.00 per year (US institutions), $100.00 per year (US students/residents), $406.00 per year (Canadian individuals), $499.00 per year (international individuals), $1024.00 per year (Canadian & international institutions), and $220.00 per year (international students/residents), $100.00 per year (Canadian & students/residents). Foreign air speed delivery is included in all *Clinics'* subscription prices. All prices are subject to change without notice. **POSTMASTER:** Send address changes to *Psychiatric Clinics of North America*, Elsevier Health Sciences Division, Subscription Customer Service, 3251 Riverport Lane, Maryland Heights, MO 63043. **Customer Service: 1-800-654-2452 (US). From outside the United States, call 1-314-447-8871. Fax: 1-314-447-8029. E-mail: journalscustomerservice-usa@elsevier.com (for print support) and journalsonlinesupport-usa@elsevier.com (for online support).**

Reprints. For copies of 100 or more, of articles in this publication, please contact the Commercial Reprints Department, Elsevier Inc., 360 Park Avenue South, New York, New York 10010-1710. Tel.: 212-633-3874, Fax: 212-633-3820, E-mail: reprints@elsevier.com.

Psychiatric Clinics of North America is covered in *MEDLINE/PubMed (Index Medicus), Current Contents/Social and Behavioral Sciences, Social Science Citation Index, Embase/Excerpta Medica,* and PsycINFO.

Contributors

CARLYLE H. CHAN, MD
Professor of Psychiatry and the Institute for Health and Equity (Bioethics and Medical Humanities); Vice Chair for Professional Development and Educational Outreach, Department of Psychiatry and Behavioral Medicine, Medical College of Wisconsin, Milwaukee, Wisconsin, USA

JUSTIN A. CHEN, MD, MPH
Assistant Professor and Co-Director of Medical Student Education in Psychiatry, Harvard Medical School, Medical Director, Outpatient Psychiatry Division, Massachusetts General Hospital, Boston, Massachusetts, USA

JOSEPH J. COOPER, MD
Associate Professor of Clinical Psychiatry, Department of Psychiatry, University of Illinois at Chicago, Chicago, Illinois, USA

ERIN M. CROCKER, MD
Department of Psychiatry, Clinical Associate Professor, Residency Training Director, University of Iowa Hospitals and Clinics, Iowa City, Iowa, USA

ELIZABETH FENSTERMACHER, MD
Department of Child Psychiatry, Cambridge Health Alliance, Cambridge Hospital, Cambridge, Massachusetts, USA; Harvard Medical School, Boston, Massachusetts, USA

JASON R. FRANK, MD, MA(Ed), FRCPC
Vice Chair, Education, Department of Emergency Medicine, University of Ottawa, Director of Specialty Education, Strategy and Standards, Royal College of Physicians and Surgeons of Canada, Ottawa, Ontario, Canada

ADRIENNE T. GERKEN, MD
Associate Program Director, Massachusetts General Hospital and McLean Hospital Adult Psychiatry Residency Program, Instructor in Psychiatry, Harvard Medical School, McLean Hospital, Belmont, Massachusetts, USA

VIKAS GUPTA, MD, MPH
South Carolina Department of Mental Health, Columbia, South Carolina, USA

ERIC S. HOLMBOE, MD
Chief Research, Milestone Development, and Evaluation Officer, Accreditation Council for Graduate Medical Education, ACGME, Chicago, Illinois, USA

VICENTA B. HUDZIAK, MD
Triple Board Resident, Department of Psychiatry and Human Behavior, The Warren Alpert Medical School of Brown University, Rhode Island Hospital, Providence, Rhode Island, USA

JEFFREY I. HUNT, MD
Professor, Department of Psychiatry and Human Behavior, The Warren Alpert Medical School of Brown University, Bradley Hospital, East Providence, Rhode Island, USA

AAVA BUSHRA JAHAN, BS
Depression Clinical and Research Program, Massachusetts General Hospital, Boston, Massachusetts, USA

A. LEE LEWIS, MD
Associate Professor, Division Director of Child and Adolescent Psychiatry, Program Director of Child and Adolescent Training, Psychiatry Clerkship Director for College of Medicine, College of Medicine, Medical University of South Carolina, Department of

Psychiatry and Behavioral Sciences, Medical University of South Carolina, Charleston, South Carolina, USA

REGINA M. LONGLEY, BA
Department of Psychiatry, Massachusetts General Hospital, Boston, Massachusetts, USA

JOHN LUO, MD
Health Sciences Clinical Professor of Psychiatry, University of California, Irvine, School of Medicine, Orange, California, USA

AUSTIN McCADDEN
Medical Student, College of Medicine, Medical University of South Carolina, Charleston, South Carolina, USA

SHANNON R. McGUE
Medical Student, College of Medicine, Medical University of South Carolina, Isle of Palms, South Carolina, USA

CHRISTINE M. PELIC, MD
Assistant Professor, Ralph H. Johnson VA Medical Center, College of Medicine, Department of Psychiatry and Behavioral Sciences, Medical University of South Carolina, Charleston, South Carolina, USA

CHRISTOPHER G. PELIC, MD
Professor, Associate Dean for GME Outreach, Medical Director for Telepsychiatry, College of Medicine, Department of Psychiatry and Behavioral Sciences, Medical University of South Carolina, Charleston, South Carolina, USA

DIANA M. ROBINSON, MD
Department of Psychiatry, Parkland Hospital, UT Southwestern Medical School, Dallas, Texas, USA

THEODORE A. STERN, MD
Chief Emeritus, Avery D. Weisman Psychiatry Consultation Service, Ned H. Cassem Professor of Psychiatry in the Field of Psychosomatic Medicine/Consultation, Harvard Medical School, Director, Thomas P. Hackett Center for Scholarship in Psychosomatic Medicine, Massachusetts General Hospital, Boston, Massachusetts, USA

NHI-HA TRINH, MD, MPH
Assistant Professor and Associate Director, Hinton Society, Harvard Medical School, Director, Psychiatry Center for Diversity, Massachusetts General Hospital, Boston, Massachusetts, USA

ROOPMA WADHWA, MD, MHA
South Carolina Department of Mental Health, Columbia, South Carolina, USA

ASHLEY E. WALKER, MD
Associate Professor, Department of Psychiatry, University of Oklahoma School of Community Medicine, Tulsa, Oklahoma, USA

ERIC R. WILLIAMS, MD
University of South Carolina School of Medicine, Columbia, South Carolina, USA

JOHN Q. YOUNG, MD, MPP, PhD
Professor and Vice Chair for Education, Department of Psychiatry, Donald and Barbara Zucker School of Medicine at Hofstra/Northwell and Zucker Hillside Hospital at Northwell Health, Glen Oaks, New York, USA

Contents

There is a robust literature on learning styles. This literature rests on 3 assumptions: (1) Individuals have a preference for a particular style of learning, (2) Individuals learn better using their preferred style, and (3) Teachers should adjust their teaching to accommodate their learner's style. One benefit of understanding learning styles is to encourage in-depth learning. This article outlines commonly used learning styles and provides a literature review on the 3 assumptions. The authors conclude that although there is some evidence for learning styles, there is little justification for adjusting teaching methods to match individual styles.

Given the significant, persistent health care inequities encountered by minority populations, health care organizations and training programs have sought to incorporate cultural competency training initiatives. However, the variety of pedagogical models demonstrate the current lack of a uniform standardized curriculum. Limitations of knowledge-based cultural competence initiatives have resulted in a shift toward attitude- and behavior-based "cultural humility." Cultural humility, the ability to maintain an interpersonal stance that is open In relation to aspects of cultural identity that are most important to the patient, expands on cultural competence, which is essential to improving patient care in mental health care settings.

Simulation-based medical education (SBME) provides experiential learning for medical trainees without any risk of harm to patients. Simulation is now included in most medical school and residency curricula. In psychiatric education, simulation programs are rapidly expanding and innovating. Major applications of SBME in psychiatry include achieving close observation of trainees with patients, preparing trainees for unstable patient scenarios, and exposing trainees to a broader range of psychopathology. This review article covers the history of SBME, simulation modalities, current use of SBME in psychiatry, a case study from one institution, and recommendations for incorporating simulation in psychiatry education.

Learning is no longer constrained to the classroom or lecture hall. Today's students expect teaching to be available 24/7 and on whatever device they own and to be interactive and engaging. Educators need to become familiar with computer-based teaching tools and learn how to implement them or risk losing their audience. Use of these tools is not merely converting the medium, say from a VHS (video home system) tape to a YouTube stream, but incorporating the features of the educational tools to facilitate active learning. Social media has become a force in the educational arena, providing a foundational framework.

Lecture presentations may first be improved by thoughtfully reflecting on how learners might best absorb the material, considering the intended audience and focusing on the essential information to be delivered. The addition of slides should augment the presentation, not draw attention away from it. Slides should contain a minimum of verbiage and bullet points. Visual images may enhance the talk. Paying attention to the style of delivery will also aid in getting the message across.

Adapting teaching to the clinical setting is most successful when the teacher and trainee are able to work alongside of each other allowing the cognitive apprenticeship model to be embraced. Six tools of experiential learning as components of this framework are described including scaffolding, modeling, coaching/supervision, articulation, reflection, and exploration. These tools provide useful guidance for supervisors to teach in clinical settings. Inherent in this process is the concept of validation of the trainees and includes the importance of supervisors cultivating nonjudgmental acceptance of themselves. Optimal teaching and learning in the clinical environment requires investment of time and resources.

Although there is debate about the importance of a strong foundation in psychotherapy for psychiatrists, the literature provides ample evidence of the positive impact on patient care outcomes when psychiatrists are competent to provide this important form of treatment. Despite financial pressures and increases in managed care posing a threat to the maintenance of psychotherapy as a core skillset for psychiatrists, psychotherapy training should not only be maintained within psychiatry residency training but should in fact be given a renewed focus and priority within training programs.

Medical education programs are failing to meet the health needs of patients and communities. Misalignments exist on multiple levels, including content (what trainees learn), pedagogy (how trainees learn), and culture (why trainees learn). To address these challenges effectively, competency-based assessment (CBA) for psychiatric medical education must simultaneously produce life-long learners who can self-regulate their own growth and trustworthy processes that determine and accelerate readiness for independent practice. The key to effectively doing so is situating assessment within a carefully designed system with several, critical, interacting components: workplace-based assessment, ongoing faculty development, learning analytics, longitudinal coaching, and fit-for-purpose clinical competency committees.

Effective feedback is critical to medical education in that it promotes learning and ensures that benchmark learning objectives are achieved. Yet the nature of and response to feedback is variable. In this article, the authors provide a comprehensive review of the effective feedback literature. Namely, they discuss the various approaches to feedback, their advantages and disadvantages, as well as barriers to providing effective feedback. Finally, they offer suggestions for steps both the feedback giver and receiver can take to foster a culture of successful feedback in an academic and clinical setting.

Multiple-choice tests are the most used method of assessment in medical education. However, there is limited literature in medical education and psychiatry to inform the best practices in writing good-quality multiple-choice questions. Moreover, few physicians and psychiatrists have received training and have experience in writing them. This article highlights the strategies in writing high-quality multiple-choice items and discusses some common flaws that can impact validity and reliability of the assessment examinations.

Narrative medicine is a patient-centered educational approach that promotes humanistic engagement of medical practitioners; it offers a unique framework for understanding medical encounters and promotes empathic connections through enhancement of observation, listening, and reflection. The andragogy of narrative medicine uniquely engages adult learners and may enhance academic learning. This article explores the evidence for narrative medicine and discusses its unique applications and potential within psychiatry. An adaptable narrative medicine curriculum is proposed for use in a 4-year psychiatric residency curriculum to allow for easy adoption of narrative medicine as an underutilized best educational practice.

Many careers are available to psychiatrist-educators, and residents should learn about these pathways in addition to developing a core set of teaching skills regardless of their intended career trajectory. Clinician-Educator Programs offer structured opportunities for residents to explore advanced concepts, practice teaching skills, pursue scholarship, and receive mentorship in medical education. Women and persons from minority groups, particularly people of color and gender-diverse individuals, have long been passed over in the promotions process, and correction of these inequities is essential to creating a robust workforce of clinician-educators.

Psychiatric education has struggled to move past dualistic notions separating mind from brain, and embrace the field's identity as a clinical neuroscience discipline. To modernize our educational systems, we must integrate neuroscience perspectives into every facet of our clinical work. To do this effectively, neuroscience education should be clinically relevant, informed by adult learning theory, and tailored to the individualized needs of learners. Classic neuropsychiatry skills can help us better understand our patients' brain function at the bedside. Integrating neuroscience perspectives alongside the other rich perspectives in psychiatry will help trainees appreciate the relevance of neuroscience to modern medical practice.

In the early twentieth century, the medical profession focused on the development of specialties and specialty/subspecialty training. Parallel to this development was the establishment of certifying boards, which can evaluate and attest to a physician's mastery of a set of knowledge and skills; the goal is to provide assurance to patients and the public of a certain guarantee of quality of care. In the early decades of "board certification," the examination was a one-time, relatively high-stakes process that assessed knowledge, and often certain skills and clinical reasoning.

With the adoption of competency-based medical education, assessment has shifted from traditional classroom domains of knows and knows how to the workplace domain of doing. This workplace-based assessment has 2 purposes; assessment of learning (summative feedback) and the assessment for learning (formative feedback). What the trainee does becomes the basis for identifying growth edges and determining readiness for advancement and ultimately independent practice. High-quality workplace-based assessment programs require thoughtful choices about the framework of assessment, the tools themselves, the platforms used, and the contexts in which the assessments take place, with an emphasis on direct observation.

PSYCHIATRIC CLINICS OF NORTH AMERICA

SERIES OF RELATED INTEREST

Child and Adolescent Psychiatric Clinics of North America
https://www.childpsych.theclinics.com/

Neurologic Clinics
https://www.neurologic.theclinics.com/

THE CLINICS ARE AVAILABLE ONLINE!
Access your subscription at:
www.theclinics.com

Preface

The *Psychiatric Clinics of North America* Special Issue on Medical Education

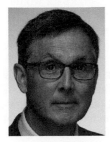 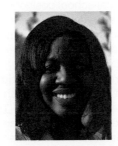

Robert J. Boland, MD   Hermioni L. Amonoo, MD, MPP
Editors

Medical education is an odd endeavor. Unlike much of the rest of education, it is usually not led by educators, but by physicians.[1] Most physician educators are experts in their clinical fields but have little formal pedagogical training.[1–4] It is not an exaggeration to assume that most medical school professors would not be permitted to teach at their children's primary schools.

The field of medical education has grown in fits and starts.[5] In the 1800s, medical schools were unregulated with no required curricula. A few high-quality, university-based medical schools, such as Johns Hopkins, Harvard, and Yale, existed, but most had no affiliation with higher-learning medical institutions.[6] Alarmed by the absence of formal medical education curricula or requirements, the American Medical Association, in 1908, asked the Carnegie Foundation for the Advancement of Teaching to survey the state of American medical education.[7] The Carnegie Foundation chose Abraham Flexner, an American educator, to lead this charge. Flexner was a curious choice. Before his appointment, he had never set foot in a medical school and had no advanced degrees. Flexner was a schoolteacher running a private school with a reputation for education reform. He had already written a best-selling critique of higher education, which advocated for smaller class sizes, fewer lectures, and more hands-on teaching. He also argued for less emphasis on research success as a criterion for faculty promotion in favor of teaching skills. Flexner applied this same critical eye to medical education. He concluded that as bad as colleges were, medical schools were worse. Flexner released his report in 1910, entitled, "Medical Education in the United States and Canada, a Report to the Carnegie Foundation for the Advancement of Teaching, Bulletin Number 4," which is better known as "The Flexner Report."[7–9] He made many bold recommendations, including

Psychiatr Clin N Am 44 (2021) xiii–xvii
https://doi.org/10.1016/j.psc.2021.03.007
0193-953X/21/© 2021 Published by Elsevier Inc.

to close all medical schools not associated with universities, standardize the medical school curriculum, incorporate laboratory and bedside learning, use a scientific approach to medicine, and expose students to properly trained role models.[10] He was incredibly passionate about this last recommendation, saying that medical school faculty should be "true university teachers, barred from all but charity practice, in the interest of teaching."

The modern medical school is, mostly, a result of Flexner's recommendations articulated in the Flexner report.[11] There were downsides to this overhaul of medical education, though. Unfortunately, the resulting closure of medical schools and the reciprocal decrease in available medical school positions created barriers for women and individuals from minority groups to become physicians for decades to come.[11,12] Still, the overall result was a dramatic increase in the quality of medical education in North America, launching the United States from its European forbearers' shadow into a center for preeminent medical science.

In this century, we have begun to reassess medical education again.[10,13] Flexner's emphasis on medical science may have focused too much on the rational while deemphasizing the art of medicine and medical humanism.[14] This and other concerns resulted in a consortium of stakeholders who formed an independent international commission with funding from the Gates and Rockefeller foundations and the China Medical Board. Chaired by Julio Frenk, former Dean of the Harvard TH Chan School of Public Health, this commission published recommendations in 2010 to transform the existing medical teaching methods, 100 years after the Flexner report.[15] This new commission emphasized competency-based assessments,[16] integrating clinical experiences earlier in the medical training process,[17] teaching social sciences with the basic and clinical sciences,[18] and emphasizing interprofessional educational experiences. The commission also called for more attention to helping students develop professional identities, including addressing medical ethics, professionalism,[19] and the "hidden curriculum."[20]

Despite many reforms and proposals for medical education in the twenty-first century, medical educators mostly employ teaching methods grounded in a behavioral approach, where the teacher provides the stimulus for learning and the consequences.[21] The goal of medical education has been to get the correct answer on a test or during clinical rounds. However, educators are now exploring newer models, such as social learning, where the learner moves from a passive recipient to an active participant in the learning relationship.[21] Similarly, constructivist learning theories elevate the learner to be the primary learning agent, drawing from novel experiences to build on their existing knowledge. Some critics of the newer teaching methods in medical education suggest that we are throwing out the old for the new. These critics are concerned that we too quickly insist on the approach du jour, such as team-based learning, over time-tested methods, like lectures.[22] Ultimately, we think that the ideal medical education program is multimodal, making the best use of various educational approaches.

Graduate medical education harbors its inherent challenges, most of the earlier work and proposals for transforming medical education have focused on undergraduate medical education. While some best practice teaching methods transcend different medical specialties, multiple factors (eg, content, competency requirements for procedural specialties, length of training, an exponential increase in evidence-based clinical care, technological advancements) make graduate medical education challenging to reform.[23] Psychiatric education has evolved over the past 2 centuries, owing to advances in neuroscience,[24] assessment methods, and therapeutics.[25,26] Efforts aimed at assessing current pedagogy for training astute psychiatric clinicians grounded in the most recent evidence in the field with the ability to tailor their care for diverse patients are warranted.[27] This issue of the *Psychiatric Clinics of North America* attempts to provide an up-to-date summary of current techniques, theories, and approaches emphasized in medical education. Although one might wish for a systematic approach covering all aspects of theory, practice, assessment, and research, the reality is less organized. The evidence is evolving, and different fields and specialties in medicine are advancing at different rates.[28] Thus, rather than supply a comprehensive report on medical education, we highlight a few key areas from various psychiatric medical education experts.

Most of the articles focus on practical skills, emphasizing educational innovations that we hope would help our readers. For example, our authors discuss how to improve our presentations, incorporate computer-based teaching, give effective feedback, and use simulations. We also consider the educators' challenges and opportunities for teaching specific subjects or in various settings, such as the clinical setting, psychotherapy training, and teaching neuroscience. We also discuss some often-neglected psychiatric education issues, including educational theory as it applies to learning styles, incorporating narrative techniques, and integrating cultural sensitivity into teaching. Assessment remains a challenge in education, and we include articles on competency-based assessments, how to write quality multiple-choice questions, and how to advance workplace-based assessments. Finally, we also discuss fostering educational careers and encouraging lifelong learning.

While this is issue is not all-encompassing, we hope that these articles will be practical and useful, inspiring a continued exploration of psychiatric education in more depth.

Robert J. Boland, MD
The Menninger Clinic
Department of Psychiatry and
Behavioral Sciences
Baylor College of Medicine
Houston, TX, USA

Hermioni L. Amonoo, MD, MPP
Department of Psychiatry
Brigham and Women's Hospital
Harvard Medical School
Boston, MA, USA

E-mail addresses:
rboland@menninger.edu (R.J. Boland)
hermioni_amonoo@dfci.harvard.edu (H.L. Amonoo)

REFERENCES

1. Steinert Y, Mann K, Centeno A, et al. A systematic review of faculty development initiatives designed to improve teaching effectiveness in medical education: BEME Guide No. 8. Med Teach 2006;28(6):497–526.

2. Whitcomb ME. The medical school's faculty is its most important asset. Acad Med 2003;78(2):117–8.

3. Searle NS, Hatem CJ, Perkowski L, et al. Why invest in an educational fellowship program? Acad Med 2006;81(11):936–40.

4. Turner TL, Ward MA, Palazzi DL, et al. Value placed on formal training in education by pediatric department chairs and residency program directors. J Grad Med Educ 2011;3(4):558–61.
5. Densen P. Challenges and opportunities facing medical education. Trans Am Clin Climatol Assoc 2011;122:48–58.
6. Verduin ML, Boland RJ, Guthrie TM. New directions in medical education related to psychiatry. Int Rev Psychiatry 2013;25(3):338–46.
7. Beck AH. STUDENTJAMA. The Flexner report and the standardization of American medical education. JAMA 2004;291(17):2139–40.
8. Flexner A. Medical education in the United States and Canada. From the Carnegie Foundation for the Advancement of Teaching, Bulletin Number Four, 1910. Bull World Health Organ 2002;80(7):594–602.
9. Barzansky B. Abraham Flexner and the era of medical education reform. Acad Med 2010;85(9 suppl):S19–25.
10. Irby DM, Cooke M, O'Brien BC. Calls for reform of medical education by the Carnegie Foundation for the Advancement of Teaching: 1910 and 2010. Acad Med 2010;85(2):220–7.
11. Steinecke A, Terrell C. Progress for whose future? The impact of the Flexner Report on medical education for racial and ethnic minority physicians in the United States. Acad Med 2010;85(2):236–45.
12. Freeman BK, Landry A, Trevino R, et al. Understanding the leaky pipeline: perceived barriers to pursuing a career in medicine or dentistry among underrepresented-in-medicine undergraduate students. Acad Med 2016;91(7):987–93.
13. Cooke M, Irby DM, Sullivan W, et al. American medical education 100 years after the Flexner report. N Engl J Med 2006;355(13):1339–44.
14. Duffy TP. The Flexner Report–100 years later. Yale J Biol Med 2011;84(3):269–76.
15. Frenk J, Chen L, Bhutta ZA, et al. Health professionals for a new century: transforming education to strengthen health systems in an interdependent world. Lancet 2010;376(9756):1923–58.
16. Frank JR, Snell LS, Cate OT, et al. Competency-based medical education: theory to practice. Med Teach 2010;32(8):638–45.
17. Wenrich MD, Jackson MB, Wolfhagen I, et al. What are the benefits of early patient contact?—A comparison of three preclinical patient contact settings. BMC Med Educ 2013;13:80.
18. Tabatabaei Z, Yazdani S, Sadeghi R. Barriers to integration of behavioral and social sciences in the general medicine curriculum and recommended strategies to overcome them: a systematic review. J Adv Med Educ Prof 2016;4(3):111–21.
19. Ludmerer KM. Instilling professionalism in medical education. JAMA 1999;282(9):881–2.
20. Lempp H, Seale C. The hidden curriculum in undergraduate medical education: qualitative study of medical students' perceptions of teaching. BMJ 2004;329(7469):770–3.
21. Badyal DK, Singh T. Learning theories: the basics to learn in medical education. Int J Appl Basic Med Res 2017;7(suppl 1):S1–3.
22. Guze PA. Using technology to meet the challenges of medical education. Trans Am Clin Climatol Assoc 2015;126:260–70.
23. Shelton PG, Corral I, Kyle B. Advancements in undergraduate medical education: meeting the challenges of an evolving world of education, healthcare, and technology. Psychiatr Q 2017;88(2):225–34.
24. Ebaugh FG. The evolution of psychiatric education. Am J Psychiatry 1969;126(1):97–100.

25. Benjamin S, Travis MJ, Cooper JJ, et al. Neuropsychiatry and neuroscience education of psychiatry trainees: attitudes and barriers. Acad Psychiatry 2014; 38(2):135–40.
26. Ross DA, Arbuckle MR, Travis MJ, et al. An integrated neuroscience perspective on formulation and treatment planning for posttraumatic stress disorder: an educational review. JAMA Psychiatry 2017;74(4):407–15.
27. Ross DA, Travis MJ, Arbuckle MR. The future of psychiatry as clinical neuroscience: why not now? JAMA Psychiatry 2015;72(5):413–4.
28. Gishen K, Ovadia S, Arzillo S, et al. The current format and ongoing advances of medical education in the United States. J Craniofac Surg 2014;25(1):35–8.

Types of Learners

Robert J. Boland, MD[a],*, Hermioni L. Amonoo, MD, MPP[b]

KEYWORDS

- Learning theory • Learning styles • Pedagogy • Teaching methods

KEY POINTS

- Students have a preferential learning style.
- A student's learning style affects their motivation to learn.
- Teaching methods can be adjusted to foster more in-depth learning.

INTRODUCTION

Optimal and impactful teaching involves more than effective teaching methods and requires a nuanced understanding of how people learn. Hence, modern teaching approaches have devoted and emphasized an understanding of learning styles. There are no standard definitions for learning styles. However, we define learning styles as preferences for how learners collect, assimilate, organize, and store information.

Learning styles rest on 3 assumptions, as follows: (1) The individuals have a preference for a particular style, one that they were likely born with; (2) That individuals learn better when they use that style; and (3) When teachers match their teaching to a preferred learning style, their students learn better.

Many examples of learning styles derive from educational, cognitive, and personality theories, and a comprehensive listing is beyond the scope of this review. Although some experts categorize learning styles based on their assumptions that learning styles are constitutionally based and fixed, others categorize learning styles based on the assumption that they are flexible and reflect personal preferences rather than actual learning ability.

For this article, the authors oversimplify the approaches into the 3 following categories: neurocognitive approaches, personality-based approaches, and metacognitive approaches. Neurocognitive approaches consider how our senses assimilate information and what we do with it. Personality-based approaches rely on theories of personality and how they influence the learning process. Metacognitive approaches consider the role of our motivations and strategies in the learning process.

---

[a] The Menninger Clinic and The Department of Psychiatry, Baylor College of Medicine, Houston, TX, USA; [b] Department of Psychiatry, Brigham and Women's Hospital, Harvard Medical School, Boston, MA, USA
* Corresponding author.
E-mail address: rboland@menninger.edu

Psychiatr Clin N Am 44 (2021) 141–148
https://doi.org/10.1016/j.psc.2020.12.001
0193-953X/21/© 2021 Elsevier Inc. All rights reserved.

The many models and approaches can be loosely grouped in each category. Here, the authors choose 1 example for each to illustrate a given category.

NEUROCOGNITIVE EXAMPLE: THE VISUAL, AUDITORY, AND KINESTHETIC/VISUAL, AUDITORY, READING, AND KINESTHETIC MODEL

The VAK model, later renamed the VARK model, was developed by Neil Fleming, a teacher in New Zealand.[1] The name is an acronym for what he believed were the primary modes of learning: visual, auditory, and kinesthetic (**Fig. 1**). The meaning of each is mostly self-explanatory: learning by looking, listening, and doing. The "R" for "reading" was later added to divide visual into the 2 categories of graphic learners: learning by looking at pictures and learning through reading.

The VARK model is, in part, based on Howard Gardner's[2] theory of multiple intelligences. Gardner proposed that there is no "general intelligence" but various intelligences. He defined "intelligence" functionally, as the ability to solve a problem or create something of value to one's culture. He identified several types of intelligence, including linguistic, musical, spatial, and kinesthetic. Thus, a person can be "smart" in one of several ways: they might be "book smart," "math smart," "musically smart," or "body smart." This theory has face validity. An athlete on the basketball court is manipulating an enormous amount of information, assessing that information, and using this to make split-second decisions. Masters of the sport can rightly be called geniuses; however, their ingenuity seems different from that of the master scholar, methodically working at a computer, carefully analyzing a text.

Gardner also believed that these types of intelligence were innate, and although he never intended them as a substrate for teaching methods, the VARK model is an example of 1 approach that applies the Gardner theory to education. The presumption is that, to maximize learning, we should first understand which type of learning a student is most proficient, and adapt teaching to that approach. For example, some students may learn best by reading, others by listening, others by watching, and others by self-practice.

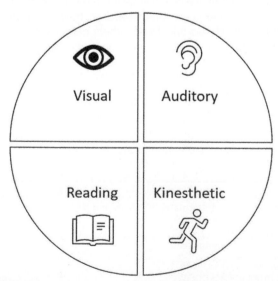

Fig. 1. The VARK model.

PERSONALITY-BASED APPROACHES: THE EXPERIENTIAL LEARNING MODEL

The Experiential Learning Model incorporates personality theory and how that affects the learning process. It was developed by David Kolb,[3] an educational theorist at Case Western University, and is also called the Kolb Model. Kolb divided learning into the 4 following stages:

First, *Concrete Experience*, in which a new experience or situation is encountered or reexperienced.

Second, *Reflective Observation*, in which the learner watches and reflects on the experience, with particular attention to any discrepancies with previous assumptions.

Third, *Abstract Conceptualization, or Theorizing,* in which thinking about the experience leads to new ideas or modifications of an existing concept.

Fourth, *Active Experimentation,* in which the learner applies the concepts to the world around them.

Kolb thought that effective learning required that a person went through all stages to truly understand a subject. However, the order one entered the series, according to Kolb, did not matter and depended on one's personality style. For example, those who preferred to begin with a concrete experience that leads to reflection had what Kolb called a "diverging" style of learning, in which they preferred to "feel" the experience first and then watch and reflect. Whereas those who like to watch and reflect to form a theory have an "assimilating style": they like to start by watching something and then thinking about it. Those who prefer to start with an abstract idea and experiment have a "converging" style: they think and then do. Those who like to experiment, which then leads to new concrete experiences, have an "accommodating style" in which they do something and then experience, or "feel" the result. Kolb believed that a person's personality determined where in the learning process a person should start. Once beginning, the learner would proceed through the stages, and only when completed would they master the topic (**Fig. 2**).

METACOGNITIVE APPROACHES: THE TRIPARTITE MODEL

The Tripartite model is metacognitive, meaning that it is primarily interested in how our motivations affect our learning style. This model was developed by Noel Entwistle, a British educational psychologist.[4] Entwistle divides styles of learning based on the learner's approach and motivation. His categories include the following: (1) Deep learning, in which the student approaches learning with intrinsic motivation and personal interest; (2) Strategic learning, in which the motivation is to be successful, such as doing well on a test; and (3) Surface learning, in which one is motivated by fear of failure. The motivation then influences the approach to learning: Deep learners want to learn everything there is about a subject; strategic learners tend to be patchier and focus on what is likely to show up on a test; and surface learners tend to rely on rote learning with a poor understanding of the subject. Unlike the other approaches, Entwistle does not suggest that these styles are innate. Instead, he assumes that, as learners, we move between learning approaches depending on our circumstances and our motivation.

EVIDENCE FOR OR AGAINST THE VARIOUS APPROACHES

Research on learning styles usually tests one of the main assumptions mentioned earlier: that individuals have a preferred style, learn better using that style, and that teaching adapted to a preferred style will produce better learning.

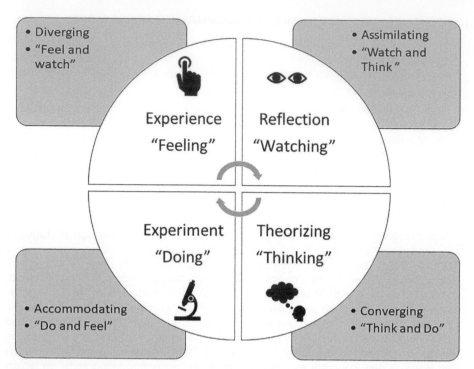

Fig. 2. The experiential learning (Kolb) model.

The bulk of research investigates whether individuals have a preferred style. Most of this research does support the hypothesis that individuals do have a preference and that preference is reasonably consistent over time. For example, Bhagat and colleagues[5] were able to group medical students into one of the VARK categories based on a questionnaire, and it had reasonable stability over time. Moreover, Meyer and colleagues,[6] studying a group of chiropractic students learning anatomy, found that most were multimodal learners with kinesthetic and visual preferences. Liew and colleagues,[7] studying an international sample of medical students, found that, when the VARK model was applied, most students had a Kinesthetic learning style. Stander and colleagues [8] reviewed the literature on learning styles in physiotherapy students and found that most had either a converging style or assimilating style. There are many other examples in the literature, and in most cases, investigators find a preferred learning style that usually remains relatively stable.

Whether individuals learn better using a preferred learning style is less clear, and there are fewer studies that focus on this question. Such a hypothesis first rests on supposing that we can divide any learning activity into a particular modality. Some investigators have tried to parse it. For example, Kumar and Chacko[9] found that teaching about learning styles helped students identify their own. The students did feel more confident in their learning, although, like many of these studies, there was no objective outcome measure. Most learning, of course, is multimodal. Some investigators suggest that even if we could restrict students to 1 approach, this is not desirable, as our students will have to learn to adjust to a multimodal world once out of training. Therefore, there is less good research in this area.

Whether adapting teaching styles to accommodate learning styles improves learning for an individual is perhaps the most critical question for teachers. Overall, there is only weak evidence for the idea that customizing teaching to preferred styles improves learning. For example, Cook and colleagues[10] used 123 medical students to determine if matching their predetermined learning style to a teaching method would affect learning outcomes. They found that their efforts did not affect the outcome. An earlier study, also lead by Cook,[11] took a similar approach with Web-based learning. Again, there was no measurable effect. Vaughn and Baker[12] also examined teacher-learner pairings with no meaningful outcomes.

In examining the literature on learning styles, Willingham and colleagues[13] points out that there are 2 main questions: do studies support the hypothesis that students with different learning styles learn better with different methods, and do students learn better with a teaching method matched to their learning style than they would have with an alternative style? In other words, it is not enough to show that different learning styles exist or that different strategies lead to different outcomes; one must show an improved outcome when matching styles to a teaching method. Willingham and colleagues give the example of an experiment in which one could divide students into visual and auditory learners. We might use 2 teaching methods, for example, watching a video or listening to a story on subsets of each group. It would not be sufficient, however, to show that learning improved when matched to the theoretically optimal teaching method. One must also show that the matched method produces better learning than the "unmatched." Thus, one might find evidence for learning styles without finding evidence that matching teaching to those styles is an effective strategy.

Although not sufficient, it would be interesting to prove either hypothesis. There are many studies on the subject and reviews of these studies, examining many populations of learners, from undergraduates to adult learners, in various disciplines.[14–27] Unfortunately, the various studies and reviews do not find evidence for either hypothesis. That is, they did not find support for the proposition that teaching to individual styles improved learning, nor did they find any evidence that matching teaching methods to a particular style produced better learning than an alternative teaching method.

Despite this lack of evidence, the idea that teachers should adapt their teaching methods to individual learning styles persists throughout all levels of education. One investigator refers to this idea as "neuromyth"[28] that persists despite the evidence.

Although there is little evidence to support adapting to individual styles, understanding learning styles is not without merit. There is robust evidence that multimodal learning improves the learning experience. Thus, rather than focusing on whether a student is a visual learner or a kinesthetic learner, understanding the VARK model may help us develop multimodal approaches that encourage students to use all the approaches.

Perhaps the most promising data are in the area of metacognition. For example, as discussed in the Tripartite model above, different types of learning are motivated by different goals. This theory has good support. Studies of this approach find that although no particular approach is intrinsic to a learner, the learner's motivation can influence the learning strategy. For example, Ferguson and colleagues[29] did a meta-analysis of studies using the Tripartite model and found that strategic learning, learning motivated by the desire for success, was associated with academic success, whereas surface learning, learning motivated by fear of failure, was negatively associated with success.

Moreover, subsequent studies[30] continue to support that although there was no evidence that any particular approach was intrinsic to any learner; method and motivation, 2 modifiable factors, mattered. For example, Fox and colleagues,[31] using a Tripartite model, found that students could successfully modify their approach based on their current needs. However, this works in both directions. Papinczak and colleagues[32] found that first-year medical students respond to the increasing load of work by moving from a strategic to a surface learning approach. Also concerning is a series of studies from 2009 to 2011 that looked at medical students' responses to introducing a new curriculum designed to promote deeper learning.[17,18] Ultimately, their approaches failed, presumably because they focused only on modifying the curriculum without considering the students and their motivations for participating in the new curriculum. Hence, the investigators concluded that learning styles did matter, but they are complicated, hard to influence, and one size does not fit all.

DISCUSSION

The evidence suggests that rather than focusing on learning styles, we should be focusing on learning approaches. Hence, instead of adapting teaching to presumed innate learning styles, it may be more useful to understand how a teaching method might encourage a particular learning approach. If one accepts that a student can adjust their learning approach depending on the situation, the teacher may wish to create a learning environment that encourages more in-depth learning. As discussed, this is not easy. However, one can presume that an emphasis, for example, on performing well on multiple-choice tests, will encourage strategic learning, which would be the most efficient approach. If we desire deeper learning, we should then consider methods that reward such learning. It is also important to note that how students are evaluated and rewarded for their learning significantly contributes to learning approaches that students will use for a given situation. Because the evidence to support learning styles and how their incorporation into teaching methods can impact learning and educational outcomes is limited, we require more research to understand the nuanced role and impact of learning styles on learning in various teaching environments.

SUMMARY

Although there remains an interest in understanding learning styles, the evidence is limited and mixed. Learning styles do exist in that individuals usually have a preferred way to learn. However, there is little evidence that these styles are static or innate. Furthermore, the existing evidence does not support teaching using these learning styles. The primary value of understanding learning styles may be that they help teachers develop multimodal learning approaches more than in individualized approaches.

The evidence, however, for learning approaches is good, and is that we can adjust our teaching (and evaluation) to encourage deeper learning in students.

CLINICS CARE POINTS

- Academic psychiatrists are often put in educational leadership positions despite not having the educational background of other teachers. Reviewing basic educational theory can inform their practice.

- As part of educational theory, educators will encounter information on learning styles. It is not reasonable to expect that medical educators should master all aspects of these theories; however, they should understand basic principles.

- There are several popular approaches to learning styles that pervade the literature. Educators should become acquainted with these concepts and the limitations and evidence supporting each theory.

- Having a general acquaintance with some of the learning theories can help the educator to develop a multimodal approach to teaching. This understanding will help foster more in-depth learning.

- The goal for every medical educator is to help produce excellent doctors. Incorporating learning theories, while avoiding being distracted by some of the "neuromyths" that surround some of these, can help the educator achieve this goal.

DISCLOSURE

The authors have nothing to disclose.

REFERENCES

1. Prithishkumar IJ, Michael SA. Understanding your student: using the VARK model. J Postgrad Med 2014;60(2):183–6.
2. Gardner H. The theory of multiple intelligences. Ann Dyslexia 1987;37(1):19–35.
3. Fewster-Thuente L, Batteson TJ. Kolb's experiential learning theory as a theoretical underpinning for interprofessional education. J Allied Health 2018;47(1):3–8.
4. Entwistle N, Ramsden P, Ramsden P. Understanding student learning (Routledge revivals). Routledge 2015. https://doi.org/10.4324/9781315718637.
5. Bhagat A, Vyas R, Singh T. Students awareness of learning styles and their perceptions to a mixed method approach for learning. Int J Appl Basic Med Res 2015;5(Suppl 1):S58–65.
6. Meyer AJ, Stomski NJ, Innes SI, et al. VARK learning preferences and mobile anatomy software application use in pre-clinical chiropractic students. Anat Sci Educ 2016;9(3):247–54.
7. Liew S-C, Sidhu J, Barua A. The relationship between learning preferences (styles and approaches) and learning outcomes among pre-clinical undergraduate medical students. BMC Med Educ 2015;15:44.
8. Stander J, Grimmer K, Brink Y. Learning styles of physiotherapists: a systematic scoping review. BMC Med Educ 2019;19(1):2.
9. Kumar LR, Chacko TV. Using appreciative inquiry to help students identify strategies to overcome handicaps of their learning styles. Educ Health (Abingdon) 2012;25(3):160–4.
10. Cook DA, Thompson WG, Thomas KG, et al. Lack of interaction between sensing-intuitive learning styles and problem-first versus information-first instruction: a randomized crossover trial. Adv Health Sci Educ Theory Pract 2009;14(1):79–90.
11. Cook DA, Gelula MH, Dupras DM, et al. Instructional methods and cognitive and learning styles in web-based learning: report of two randomised trials. Med Educ 2007;41(9):897–905.
12. Vaughn LM, Baker RC. Do different pairings of teaching styles and learning styles make a difference? Preceptor and resident perceptions. Teach Learn Med 2008;20(3):239–47.
13. Willingham DT, Hughes EM, Dobolyi DG. The scientific status of learning styles theories. Teach Psychol 2015;42(3):266–71.
14. Tarver SG, Dawson MM. Modality preference and the teaching of reading: a review. J Learn Disabil 1978;11(1):5–17.
15. Arter JA, Jenkins JR. Differential diagnosis—prescriptive teaching: a critical appraisal. Rev Educ Res 1979;49(4):517–55.
16. Kampwirth TJ, Bates M. Modality preference and teaching method: a review of the research. Acad Ther 1980;15(5):597–605.

17. Kavale KA, Forness SR. Substance over style: assessing the efficacy of modality testing and teaching. Except Child 1987;54(3):228–39.
18. Snider VE. Learning styles and learning to read: a critique. Remedial Spec Educ 1992;13(1):6–18.
19. Stahl SA. A critique of learning styles. Am Educ 1999;23:1–5.
20. Kavale KA, LeFever GB. Dunn and Dunn model of learning-style preferences: critique of Lovelace meta-analysis. J Educ Res 2007;101(2):94–7.
21. Mammen JMV, Fischer DR, Anderson A, et al. Learning styles vary among general surgery residents: analysis of 12 years of data. J Surg Educ 2007;64(6): 386–9.
22. Pashler H, McDaniel M, Rohrer D, et al. Learning styles: concepts and evidence. Psychol Sci Public Interest 2008;9(3):105–19.
23. Rohrer D, Pashler H. Learning styles: where's the evidence? Med Educ 2012; 46(7):634–5.
24. Wilkinson T, Boohan M, Stevenson M. Does learning style influence academic performance in different forms of assessment? J Anat 2014;224(3):304–8.
25. Griffiths C, İnceçay G. Styles and style-stretching: how are they related to successful learning? J Psycholinguist Res 2016;45(3):599–613.
26. İlçin N, Tomruk M, Yeşilyaprak SS, et al. The relationship between learning styles and academic performance in TURKISH physiotherapy students. BMC Med Educ 2018;18(1):291.
27. Husmann PR, O'Loughlin VD. Another nail in the coffin for learning styles? Disparities among undergraduate anatomy students' study strategies, class performance, and reported VARK learning styles. Anat Sci Educ 2019;12(1):6–19.
28. Newton PM. The learning styles myth is thriving in higher education. Front Psychol 2015;6:1908.
29. Ferguson E, James D, Madeley L. Factors associated with success in medical school: systematic review of the literature. BMJ 2002;324(7343):952–7.
30. Feeley A-M, Biggerstaff DL. Exam success at undergraduate and graduate-entry medical schools: is learning style or learning approach more important? A critical review exploring links between academic success, learning styles, and learning approaches among school-leaver entry ("traditional") and graduate-entry ("nontraditional") medical students. Teach Learn Med 2015;27(3):237–44.
31. Fox RA, McManus IC, Winder BC. The shortened study process questionnaire: an investigation of its structure and longitudinal stability using confirmatory factor analysis. Br J Educ Psychol 2001;71(Pt 4):511–30.
32. Papinczak T, Young L, Groves M, et al. Effects of a metacognitive intervention on students' approaches to learning and self-efficacy in a first year medical course. Adv Health Sci Educ Theory Pract 2008;13(2):213–32.

Moving from Cultural Competence to Cultural Humility in Psychiatric Education

Nhi-Ha Trinh, MD, MPH[a],*, Aava Bushra Jahan, BS[b], Justin A. Chen, MD, MPH[c]

KEYWORDS

- Culture • Psychiatry • Competency • Humility • Health care • Psychiatry residency
- Training

KEY POINTS

- Cultural influences impact patients' experience of and interactions with psychiatry.
- The *Diagnostic and Statistical Manual of Mental Disorders*, 5th edition, has multiple tools to incorporate culture in psychiatric clinical practice.
- Larger sociocultural systems (race, sexuality, historical precedent, the cultures of medicine and psychiatry) must be considered in the modern-day practice of psychiatry.

INTRODUCTION

The United States continues to become increasingly diverse. The US Census Bureau projects a 90% increase in racial and ethnic minorities by 2050,[1,2] which will result in a "majority minority" nation, with no racial/ethnic group exceeding 50% of the total population.[3] This cultural, socioeconomic, and linguistic diversity has the potential to foster progressive ideals and the construction of a more vibrant and culturally inclusive society. However, minority groups continue to encounter persistent structural barriers and inequalities, which impede access to quality health care.[4] In the context of debilitating psychiatric conditions, individuals from minority groups experience lower rates of remission and higher rates of chronic impairment, leading to a disproportionately higher burden of mental health disparities.[5]

Culture is a dynamic and ever-evolving construct, encompassing "the customary beliefs, social norms, and material traits of a racial, religious, or social group."[6] Culture

[a] Hinton Society, Harvard Medical School, Psychiatry Center for Diversity, Massachusetts General Hospital, One Bowdoin Square, Sixth Floor, Boston, MA 02113, USA; [b] Depression Clinical & Research Program, Massachusetts General Hospital, One Bowdoin Square, Sixth Floor, Boston, MA 02114, USA; [c] Harvard Medical School, Outpatient Psychiatry Division, Massachusetts General Hospital, 15 Parkman Street, WACC 812, Boston, MA, USA
* Corresponding author.
E-mail address: NTRINH@mgh.harvard.edu

Psychiatr Clin N Am 44 (2021) 149–157
https://doi.org/10.1016/j.psc.2020.12.002
0193-953X/21/© 2020 Elsevier Inc. All rights reserved.

psych.theclinics.com

Abbreviations	
DSM	*Diagnostic and Statistical Manual of Mental Disorders*
PGY	postgraduate year

is not a finite collection of ethnographic information, nor is it fixed or homologous to distinct individuals or communities. It provides a flexible lens through which individuals interpret culturally relevant information and construct hierarchies of shared objectives and principles.[6] Cultural variations in the perception and expression of psychiatric syndromes may contribute to diverse symptomatology, clinical assessment, and treatment trajectories.[7,8]

The impediments encountered by racial, ethnic, religious, and sexual minorities within the mental health care system are multifaceted.[9] Informed knowledge regarding the cultural context underlying distinct emotional, cognitive, and behavioral expressions is essential for competent health care delivery.[10] Providers must be adequately equipped to comprehend the meaning and significance of culturally circumscribed information beyond the application of traditional psychotherapeutic interventions. A lack of understanding regarding the unique perspectives of culturally distinct individuals and communities may adversely impact treatment adherence and effective therapeutic transactions in psychiatric settings.[11]

DEFINITION OF CULTURAL COMPETENCY

Psychosocial factors and intersecting identities influence a given individual's cultural characteristics.[12] The multifaceted components of culture contribute to a diverse spectrum for any given individual, with broad-ranging implications for clinical interactions and outcomes.[11] Given this complexity, greater efforts have been made in recent decades to formally integrate cultural competency standards into professional practice guidelines and training milestones.[13] Cultural competency can be defined as "a set of congruent behaviors, attitudes, and policies that come together in a system, agency or among professionals and enable that system, agency or those professions to work effectively in cross-cultural situations."[14] These interventions address diversity and inequality on 3 distinct levels of operation—organizational, structural, and clinical. Cultural competency can therefore be understood as referring to providers' attitudes and health care systems' capacities "to function effectively within the realm of cultural beliefs, behaviors, and needs presented by the consumer and their communities."[14] Cultural competency training provides a conceptual framework for equipping health care providers in diverse settings to facilitate culturally appropriate therapeutic interactions.[15,16]

CULTURAL COMPETENCY IN HEALTH CARE

Regulatory bodies and health care institutions have mandated efforts to enhance cultural competency training in medical education.[17] In efforts to advance equity and mitigate health disparities, the Office of Minority Health published the first National Standards on Culturally and Linguistically Appropriate Services in Health and Health Care in 2000.[18] These so-called National CLAS Standards issued a recommendation to "educate and train governance, leadership, and workforce in culturally and linguistically appropriate policies and practices on an ongoing basis."[19] The American Psychiatric Association does not publish specific guidelines regarding cultural competence or practitioner awareness.[20] However, the American Psychiatric

Association guidelines for Psychiatric Assessment of Adults offers sample questions regarding the sociocultural history of patients.[21]

Additionally, the American Psychiatric Association's *Diagnostic and Statistical Manual of Mental Disorders*, 4th edition (DSM-IV), introduced the Outline for Cultural Formulation, which became increasingly operationalized with the Cultural Formulation Interview in the DSM-5.[22] The Cultural Formulation Interview provides clinicians with a systematic approach for eliciting a patient's explanatory model, with attention to 4 principle assessment domains—(1) cultural perceptions of cause, (2) context and support, (3) self-coping and past help seeking, and (4) current help seeking and developmental dimensions.[23] Instead of obtaining cultural information via a symptom checklist, this semistructured, 16-item questionnaire directly examines the influence of sociocultural factors on diagnostic assessment and treatment outcomes.[24]

Accrediting bodies for allopathic undergraduate and graduate medical institutions, including the Liaison Committee for Medical Education and the Accreditation Council on Graduate Medical Education, have incorporated the principle of cultural humility into undergraduate and medical curricula.[25,26] The Accreditation Council on Graduate Medical Education also provides supplemental guidelines for specific subspecialties.[25] The American Academy of Child and Adolescent Psychiatry developed a "Practice Parameter on Cultural Competence in Child and Adolescent Psychiatric Practice."[27] This pedagogical framework educates providers regarding a range of relevant topics, including legal and linguistic barriers to care, idiomatic expressions of distress, differential developmental trajectories and symptom presentation, intergenerational accultured stress, underlying ethnopharmacologic factors, and the history of immigration, loss, and trauma.[28,29]

CULTURAL COMPETENCY CURRICULA IN PSYCHIATRY RESIDENCY

In addition to professional guidelines and formal assessment tools, several psychiatry residency training programs have developed a range of curricula related to cultural competence.[30] We summarize a sampling these curricula and their unique features.

The Department of Psychiatry at New York University Langone Health has established a structural competency and global mental health curriculum.[31] Structural competency is "the trained ability to discern how a host of issues, defined clinically as symptoms, attitudes, or diseases, also represent the downstream implications of a number of upstream decisions about such matters as health care and food delivery systems, zoning laws, urban and rural infrastructures, medicalization, or even about the very definitions of illness and health."[32] This didactic course exposes residents to social determinants of mental health.[31,32] Trainees are provided opportunities to develop cross-cultural communication skills, attend workshops regarding national and global diversity, and actively participate in public policy engagement regarding mental health equity.[31]

The University of California, Davis offers a 4-year cultural psychiatry curriculum.[33] This pedagogical approach exposes trainees to a broad spectrum of topics regarding diversity including Ethnographies of Self, Women's, LGBTQ+, Refugee and Global Mental Health, Structural Competency, Spirituality, Psychotherapy and Trauma-Informed Care. Residents are instructed to use concrete knowledge, attitudes, and skills to formulate culturally responsive clinical practices.[34]

Columbia University offers a course on "Cultural Formulation" during postgraduate year (PGY)-2 and "Diversity and Disparity in Clinical Treatment" during PGY-3.[35] Residents are taught to address patient-specific cultural formulations, language barrier implications, culture-specific syndromes, and folk belief systems.[36]

The University of Washington investigates the impact of refugee mental health and interpreter service efficacy on clinical encounters.[37] It also emphasizes the role of religion and spirituality in mediating culturally circumscribed narratives regarding psychopathology and therapeutic interventions.

The Cultural Competency Model at Tulane University incorporates 7 core concepts, namely, explanatory models, value orientation, acculturation, family history, racial identity, social construct, and clinical encounter.[38] A critical examination of each concept is performed through academic coursework and experiential reading seminars. These concepts are applied in accordance with the Outline for Cultural Formulation to ensure appropriate diagnostic assessment and treatment outcomes.

The Cambridge Health Alliance offers an 8-week multidisciplinary seminar called "Cross Cultural Issues in Psychiatry."[39] Residents and faculty members facilitate discussions regarding the impact of health care disparities on psychopathology, in the context of diverse patient populations.

The Division of Social and Transcultural Psychiatry at McGill University uses a pedagogical training approach.[40] The curriculum comprises academic courses, clinical rotations, intensive summer programs, and annual Advanced Study Institutes. It emphasizes knowledge acquisition and the accurate interpretation of culturally circumscribed information. The curriculum provides a conceptual framework for providers to examine the intersectional influence of culture on therapeutic transactions.[41,42]

The Massachusetts General Hospital/McLean Hospital Adult Psychiatry Residency Program offers a 3-year Sociocultural Psychiatry Curriculum.[10] The curriculum integrates socioculturally informed topics such as global psychiatric epidemiology, anthropology, religion, and spirituality.[29] PGY-1 grounds residents in an attitude of cultural humility and self-reflection. PGY-2 provides foundational knowledge regarding global psychiatry, the social determinants of health, and implicit bias in health care, as well as sociocultural psychiatry. PGY-3 uses experiential workshops to address a diverse spectrum of clinical and ethical challenges associated with cross-cultural psychiatric encounters.[34]

CHALLENGES IN CULTURAL COMPETENCY EDUCATION

Cultural competency training is essential for providers operating in integrated health care settings.[29] Training curricula are applicable to practicing physicians, residents, fellows, and medical students.[34] However, the wealth of different didactic and pedagogical models described elsewhere in this article demonstrates the lack of any standardized curriculum. Existing curricula are predominantly catered toward individual institutions, and teaching strategies are tailored toward resident-centered knowledge and preparedness, patient demographics, and local community requirements.[10] Although this provides an important opportunity to adapt each training curricula program's to its local context, the resulting heterogeneity makes it difficult to develop a uniform model curriculum.[36]

Although the fundamental role of culture in psychiatry is evident, the implementation of appropriate teaching strategies remains ambiguous. A primary challenge encountered by faculty members and attendings is the lack of formal training regarding cultural competence.[40] Cultural subjects are often sensitive, and may cause offense if not facilitated carefully.[17,41] Educators may find themselves at a disadvantage relative to their trainees, who are often comparatively well-informed regarding sociocultural issues pertaining to diverse patient populations. Attempts to operationalize culture and impart concrete knowledge, learning objectives, and skills may risk tokenism.[32,43] Focusing on the cultivation of self-knowledge and culturally relevant attitudes may seem to be abstract and impractical to residents undergoing the rigor of clinical training.[36] Generalizing the multifaceted components of culture may unwittingly perpetuate racial and ethnic stereotypes and reductive perspectives regarding its influence on psychopathology and treatment outcomes.[9,10]

CULTURAL HUMILITY IN PSYCHIATRY RESIDENCY

Awareness of the limitations of knowledge-based cultural competence have resulted in a shift toward attitude-based cultural humility.[44] This approach "incorporates a health provider's commitment and active engagement in a lifelong practice of self-evaluation and self-critique within the context of the patient–provider (or health professional) relationship through patient-oriented interviewing and care."[45] Cultural humility is not an achieved destination, but rather a lifelong endeavor. Cultural humility emphasizes cross-cultural communication and sustained dedication is required to formulate therapeutic relationships between patient and provider.[1,46] Improving intercultural communication requires cultivating a "critical consciousness"[47] in which the clinical trainee reflects on how disparities in health outcomes are mediated by systemic and social structures. Cultural humility provides a conceptual framework for health care providers to increase self-awareness and reflect on the influences of personal sociocultural identities, biases, and assumptions on clinical encounters and therapeutic encounters.[48,49]

FUTURE DIRECTIONS

Recently published curricula have incorporated topics regarding ethnographically diverse populations (Native Americans, Latinx Americans, Asian Americans, and African Americans) and sexual orientations (lesbian, gay, bisexual, transgender, and queer or questioning (LGBTQ) individuals).[50] Educators have described the use of observed structured clinical examinations to assess learning outcomes in diverse health care settings.[51,52] A possible trajectory of future research could be aimed at developing video-recorded observed structured clinical examinations or computer simulation assessment tools to enhance the scalability and replicability of educational endeavors. Another direction could focus on the usefulness of multimodal treatment techniques to deliver culturally sensitive health care.[53] The inherent flexibility of teaching produces a multitude of educational topics and formats. These pedagogical tools could be used to develop nationally and publicly available databases comprising sociocultural psychiatry sessions and evaluation tools. Educators could use these materials to construct educational curricula regarding cultural sensitivity in psychiatry education.[54]

The development of a culturally sensitive and humble workforce is critical for the delivery of quality psychiatric health care.[55] As cultural influences often mediate symptoms of psychopathology,[3,4] a culturally sensitive and humble workforce is required to facilitate effective cross-cultural psychiatric interventions in integrated health care settings.[56–58]

SUMMARY

Cultural sensitivity and humility in medical education serve as an initial step toward inclusion and equity by addressing the sociocultural impediments encountered by minority populations. Cultural competence standards are aspirational and provide an integrative framework for clinical assessment through a culturally sensitive and patient-oriented lens. Research continues to demonstrate the historical and persistent

154   Trinh et al

influences of culture on symptom presentation, treatment adherence, and therapeutic outcomes. Regulatory bodies and health care institutions have increasingly mandated efforts to integrate culturally informed curricula into residency training. The development of a culturally sensitive and humble workforce is critical for the delivery of quality psychiatric health care. An improved understanding of diverse patient populations will inevitably contribute to the development of more culturally nuanced and effective educational and clinical models, aiding providers in delivering health care to a range of individuals suffering from psychiatric conditions.

CLINICS CARE POINTS

Advantages
- Regulatory and health care institution advocacy is needed for cultural competency education in psychiatry residency training.
- DSM-5 guidance provides cultural framework and tools for the diagnostic assessment and treatment of diverse patient populations.
- Training and supervision in cultural psychiatry can improve effective cross-cultural therapeutic interactions between patients and providers, potentially mitigating persistent mental health care disparities.

Disadvantages
- Currently, there is a lack of a uniform model curriculum for sociocultural education.
- Psychiatric educators themselves may lack formal, standardized training regarding cultural competence, sensitivity, and humility.
- Attempts to operationalize education on cultural topics may risk stereotyping, reductionism, and tokenism.

DISCLOSURE

The authors have nothing to disclose.

REFERENCES

1. Hook JN, Davis DE, Owen J, et al. Cultural humility: measuring openness to culturally diverse clients. J Couns Psychol 2013;60:353.
2. Colby SL, Ortman JM. Projections of the size and composition of the U.S. Population: 2014 to 2060. United States Census Bureau; 2015. p. 25–1143. Available at: https://www.census.gov/library/publications/2015/demo/p25-1143.html.
3. It's official: The U.S. is becoming a minority-majority nation. US News & World Report. Available at: https://www.usnews.com/news/articles/2015/07/06/its-official-the-us-is-becoming-a-minority-majority-nation. Accessed June 1, 2020.
4. Breslau J, Kendler KS, Su M, et al. Lifetime Risk and Persistence of Psychiatric Disorders Across Ethnic Groups in the United States. Psychol Med 2005;35(3): 317–27.
5. Safran MA, Mays RA, Huang LN, et al. Mental health disparities. Am J Public Health 2009;99(11):1962–6.
6. Definition of Culture. Merriam-Webster Dictionary. Available at: https://www.merriam-webster.com/dictionary/culture. Accessed June 1, 2020.
7. Coleman K, Stewart C, Waltzfelder BE, et al. Racial-ethnic differences in psychiatric diagnoses and treatment across 11 health care systems in the mental research network. Psychiatr Serv 2016;67(7):749–57.

8. Ballenger JC, Davidson JRT, Lecrubier Y, et al. Consensus statement on transcultural issues in depression and anxiety from the International Consensus Group on Depression and Anxiety. J Clin Psychiatry 2001;62(13):22–30.
9. Smedley BD, Stith AY, Nelson AR. Unequal treatment: confronting racial and ethnic disparities in health care. Washington (DC): National Academies Press; 2003. https://doi.org/10.17226/12875.
10. Trinh NH, Dean T. Culture and Depression: Clinical Considerations for Racial and Ethnic Minorities. In: Shapero B, Mischoulon D, Cusin C, editors. The Massachusetts General Hospital Guide to Depression. Current Clinical Psychiatry. Cham: Humana Press; 2019. https://doi.org/10.1007/978-3-319-97241-1_4.
11. Chen JA, Durham MP, Madu A, et al. Culture and Psychiatry. In: Stern TA, Freudenreich O, Smith FA, et al, editors. Massachusetts General Hospital handbook of general hospital psychiatry. 7th edition. Philadelphia: Elsevier; 2018. p. 559–68.
12. Office of the Surgeon General (US), Center for Mental Health Services (US), National Institute of Mental Health (US). Mental health: culture, race, and ethnicity: a supplement to mental health: a report of the surgeon general. Rockville (MD): Substance Abuse and Mental Health Services Administration (US); 2001. Available at: http://www.ncbi.nlm.nih.gov/books/NBK44243/.
13. Betancourt JR. Cross-cultural medical education: conceptual approaches and frameworks for evaluation. Acad Med 2003;78(6):560–9.
14. National Center for Cultural Competence: Curricula Enhancement Module Series [Internet]. Georgetown University Center for Child and Human Development. Available at: https://nccc.georgetown.edu/curricula/culturalcompetence.html. Accessed June 1, 2020.
15. Smedley BD, Stith AY, Nelson AR. et al. Interventions: cross-cultural education in the health professions. Washington (DC): National Academies Press (US); 2003;6. Available at: https://www.ncbi.nlm.nih.gov/books/NBK220364/.
16. Metzl JM, Hansen H. Structural competency: theorizing a new medical engagement with stigma and inequality. Soc Sci Med 2013;103:126–33.
17. Ambrose AJH, Lin SY, Chun MBJ. Cultural competency training requirements in graduate medical education. J Grad Med Educ 2013;5(2):227–31.
18. Culturally and Linguistically Appropriate Services. Think Cultural Health. Available at: https://thinkculturalhealth.hhs.gov/. Accessed June 1, 2020.
19. The National CLAS Standard. U.S. Department of Health and Human Services Office of Minority Health. Available at: https://minorityhealth.hhs.gov/omh/browse.aspx?lvl=2&lvlid=53.
20. American Psychiatric Association. Available at: https://www.psychiatry.org/. Accessed June 1, 2020.
21. Silverman JJ, Galanter M, Jackson-Triche M, et al. The American Psychiatric Association practice guidelines for the psychiatric evaluation of adults. Am J Psychiatry 2015;172(8):798–802.
22. Lewis-Fernández R, Aggarwal NK, Bäärnhielm S, et al. Culture and psychiatric evaluation: operationalizing cultural formulation for DSM-5. Psychiatry 2014; 77(2):130–54.
23. American Psychiatric Association. Diagnostic and statistical manual of mental disorders: DSM-IV [Internet]. 4th ed. Washington (DC): American Psychiatric Association; 1994. p. 866. Available at: http://www.psychiatryonline.com/DSMPDF/dsm-iv.pdf.
24. Lewis-Fernandez R, Aggarwal NK, Hinton L, et al. DSM-5 Handbook on the cultural formulation Interview. Arlington (VA): American Psychiatric Publishing; 2015.

25. Standards, Publications, & Notification Forms | LCME. Available at: https://lcme.org/publications/. Accessed February 1, 2020.

26. Swing SR. The ACGME outcome project: retrospective and prospective. Med Teach 2007;29(7):648–54.

27. AACAP diversity and cultural competency curriculum. American Academy of Child & Adolescent Psychiatry; 2011. Available at: https://www.aacap.org/AACAP/Resources_for_Primary_Care/Diversity_and_Cultural_Competency_Curriculum/Home.aspx.

28. Pumariega AJ, Rothe E, Mian A, et al. American Academy of Child and Adolescent Psychiatry (AACAP) Committee on Quality Issues (CQI). https://doi.org/10.1016/j.jaac.2013.06.019. Accessed June 1, 2020.

29. Pumariega AJ, Rothe E, Mian A, et al. Practice parameter for cultural competence in child and adolescent psychiatric practice. J Am Acad Child Adolesc Psychiatry 2013;52(10):1101–15.

30. Fung K, Andermann L, Zaretsky A, et al. An integrative approach to cultural competence in the psychiatric curriculum. Acad Psychiatry 2008;32:272–82.

31. NYU Psychiatry Residency Curriculum in Cultural, Structural and Global Mental Health. Psychiatry. Available at: https://med.nyu.edu/psych/education/residency-program/nyu-psychiatry-residency-curriculum-cultural-structural-and-global-mental-health. Accessed June 1, 2020.

32. Metzl JM, Hansen H. Structural competency: theorizing a new medical engagement with stigma and inequality. Soc Sci Med 2014. https://doi.org/10.1016/j.socscimed.2013.06.032.

33. Cultural Psychiatry. UCDavis Health. Available at: https://health.ucdavis.edu/psychiatry/specialties/diversity/curriculum.html. Accessed June 1, 2020.

34. Bourgois P, Holmes SM, Sue K, et al. Structural vulnerability: operationalizing the concept to address health disparities in clinical care. Acad Med 2017;92(3):299–307.

35. Neff J, Knight KR, Satterwhite S, et al. Teaching structure: a qualitative evaluation of a structural competency training for resident physicians. J Gen Intern Med 2017;32(4):430–3. Available at: https://www.ncbi.nlm.nih.gov/pubmed/27896692.

36. Corral I, Johnson TL, Shelton PH, et al. Psychiatry resident training in cultural competence: an educator's toolkit. Psychiatry Q 2017;88:295–306. Available at: https://medschool.ucsd.edu/som/psychiatry/about/Diversity/Documents/Corral2017_Article_PsychiatryResidentTrainingInCu.pdf.

37. New York State Center of Excellence for Cultural Competence. Columbia University Department of Psychiatry. [Internet]. Available at: https://www.columbiapsychiatry.org/research/research-centers/new-york-state-center-excellence-cultural-competence. Accessed June 1, 2020.

38. Kirmayer LJ. Rethinking cultural competence. Trans Psychiatry 2012;49(2):149–64.

39. UW Religion, spirituality, and culture curriculum. Available at: http://psychres.washington.edu/syllabiandreadings/rscsyllabus.asp. Accessed June 1, 2020.

40. Pena JM, Manguno-Mire G, Kinzie E, et al. Teaching cultural competence to psychiatry residents: seven core concepts and their implications for therapeutic technique. Acad Psychiatry 2016;40(2):328–36. Available at: https://www.ncbi.nlm.nih.gov/pubmed/25749919.

41. Didactic Thematic Structures and Values of the program. Cambridge Health Alliance. Available at: https://www.challiance.org/academic/adult-psychiatry-didactics. Accessed June 1, 2020.

42. Kirmayer LJ, Rousseau C, Guzder J, et al. Training clinicians in cultural psychiatry: a Canadian perspective. Acad Psychiatry 2008;32(4):313–9. Available at: https://link.springer.com/article/10.1176/appi.ap.32.4.313.

43. Kirmayer LJ, Fang K, Rousseau C, et al. Canadian Psychiatric Association Position Paper: guidelines for training in cultural psychiatry 2012. Available at: https://www.researchgate.net/publication/234008626_Guidelines_for_Training_in_Cultural_Psychiatry-Position_Paper.

44. Publisher apologises for "racist" text in medical book - BBC News. Available at: https://www.bbc.com/news/blogs-trending-41692593. Accessed February 1, 2020.

45. Gregg J, Saha S. Losing culture on the way to competence: the use and misuse of culture in medical education. Acad Med 2006;81(6):542–7.

46. Fisher-Borne M, Cain JM, Martin SL. From mastery to accountability: cultural humility as an alternative to cultural competence. Soc Work Educ 2014;34(2): 165–81.

47. Tervalon M, Murray-García J. Cultural humility versus cultural competence: a critical distinction in defining physician training outcomes in multicultural education. J Health Care Poor Underserved 1998;9(2):117–25.

48. Yeager KA, Bauer-Wu S, Hodgson N, et al. Cultural humility: essential foundation for clinical researchers. Appl Nurs Res 2013;26(4):251–6.

49. Danso R. Cultural competence and cultural humility: a critical reflection on key cultural diversity concepts. Soc Work Educ 2016. https://doi.org/10.1177/1468017316654341.

50. Chang E, Simon M, Dong X. Integrating cultural humility into health care professional education and training. Adv Health Sci Educ 2012;17:269–78.

51. Juarez JA, Marvel K, Brezinski KL, et al. Bridging the gap: a curriculum to teach residents cultural humility. Fam Med 2006;38(2):97–102.

52. The psychiatry milestone project. J Grad Med Educ 2014;6(1 Suppl 1):284–304.

53. Hodges B, Regehr G, Hanson M, et al. Validation of an objective structured clinical examination in psychiatry. Acad Med 1998;73(8):910–2.

54. Loschen EL. Using the objective structured clinical examination in a psychiatry residency. Acad Psychiatry 1993;17:95–100.

55. Gorrindo T, Baer L, Sanders KM, et al. Web-based stimulation in psychiatry residency training: a pilot study. Acad Psychiatry 2011;35:232–7.

56. Gorrindo T, Goldfarb E, Birnbaum RJ, et al. Stimulation-based ongoing professional practice evaluation in psychiatry: a novel tool for performance assessment. Jt Comm J Qual Patient Saf 2013;39(7):319–23.

57. Lokko HN, Chen JA, Parekh RI, et al. Racial and Ethnic Diversity in the US psychiatric workforce: a perspective and recommendations. Acad Psychiatry 2016; 40:898–904.

58. Simonsen K, Shim RS. Embracing diversity and inclusion in psychiatry leadership. Psychiatr Clin 2019;42(3):463–71.

The Use of Simulation in Teaching

Shannon R. McGue[a], Christine M. Pelic, MD[b,c], Austin McCadden[a], Christopher G. Pelic, MD[b],*, A. Lee Lewis, MD[b]

KEYWORDS

- Simulation • Teaching • Simulation-based medical education
- Psychiatric education • Mental health education

KEY POINTS

- Simulation-based medical education (SBME) offers meaningful experiential learning opportunities without risk to patients.
- SBME has been shown to improve outcomes at multiple translational levels.
- In psychiatric education, simulation programs are rapidly expanding and innovating, though research on outcomes is still limited.
- Simulation modalities include low-technology models (eg, anatomic models, inert mannequins), standardized patients, screen-based computer simulations, complex task trainers, high-fidelity patient simulators (eg, interactive mannequins), and virtual reality systems.

INTRODUCTION

Traditional medical education is rooted in the nineteenth-century ideology pioneered by Sir William Osler that students should learn medicine through direct patient experiences, complemented by classroom learning.[1] In a twenty-first century drive to increase experiential learning while simultaneously decreasing patient risk, simulation-based exercises have emerged as an exciting new educational tool. Simulation allows for standardization of educational experiences, which is hard to achieve in clinical settings. In addition, simulating high-risk scenarios in a safe environment can help teach crisis management skills efficiently.[2,3]

Because of these advantages, simulation-based medical education (SBME) has been widely adopted in undergraduate and graduate programs.[4] According to the Association of American Medical Colleges (AAMC), simulation is arguably the most prominent innovation in medical education in recent history.

[a] College of Medicine, Medical University of South Carolina, 96 Jonathan Lucas Street, Suite 812, MSC 623, Charleston, SC 29425, USA; [b] Department of Psychiatry and Behavioral Sciences, Medical University of South Carolina, 67 President Street, MSC 861, Charleston, SC 29425, USA; [c] Ralph H. Johnson VA Medical Center, 109 Bee Street, Charleston, SC 29401, USA
* Corresponding author.
E-mail address: pelicc@musc.edu

Psychiatr Clin N Am 44 (2021) 159–171
https://doi.org/10.1016/j.psc.2021.03.002
0193-953X/21/© 2021 Elsevier Inc. All rights reserved.

Simulation is especially helpful in psychiatric education because direct observation of patient care and immediate feedback to the trainee are difficult to achieve. Observing residents as they build rapport with the patients in their clinic panel, for example, would violate the privacy that is required for developing a psychiatrist-patient relationship and diminish trust by potentially conveying that teaching is prioritized over patient care.[5]

Selecting a simulation modality most often depends on the educational goals of the activity and the resources available. Simulation modalities can be classified into 6 major groups[5–7]:

1. Low-technology: low-cost models or mannequins used to teach basic knowledge or psychomotor skills.
2. Standardized patients (SPs): actors trained to portray patients, who can facilitate teaching and assessment of history taking, physical examination, communication skills, and professionalism.
3. Screen-based computer simulators: software for training and assessment of clinical knowledge and decision making.
4. Complex task trainers: computer-based task trainers used for high-fidelity procedural skills.
5. High-fidelity patient simulators: computer-based mannequins used for replication of complex and high-risk clinical conditions in lifelike settings.
6. Virtual reality: emerging technology that involves sensory inputs and various user receptors (eg, head tracker); may be used for a wide variety of learning and assessment purposes.

Evidence has shown that simulation has clear benefits in educational outcomes.[8–10] Areas that warrant further research include impact on patient outcomes, sustainability of simulation efforts, and cost-effectiveness of training programs.[3]

Demonstrating the effectiveness of simulation is important because there are significant costs associated with implementing and maintaining simulation in medical curricula. Purchasing and maintenance of equipment, university space, and faculty hours in the curriculum development and implementation are all costs that must be considered for each institution.[11] Evidence for effectiveness can also help overcome educational inertia, which is described as the interacting factors that lead medical schools to resist change in education.[1,12]

This article describes the history and theory of SBME, characterizes different types of simulation, and details current use of simulation in psychiatric medical education. We then present a case study performed at the Medical University of South Carolina (MUSC) and finally provide recommendations on how to incorporate simulation in psychiatric education, based on this literature review and our own experience in SBME.

HISTORY OF SIMULATION-BASED MEDICAL EDUCATION

Widespread use of simulation was adopted in other fields before the more recent boom in medical education. The military has long used simulation as a mode of preparation and training. The modern military accounted for 80% of all modeling and simulation work before the 1990s.[13]

In 1929, Edwin Albert Link invented the first flight simulator, which consisted of a fuselagelike device equipped with a cockpit and controls.[14] The US Army Air Corps purchased Link's simulator in reaction to a series of postal carrier plane accidents, and after quickly proving its worth, the simulator became a mandatory part of pilot training in many countries.[13] Other industries like the space program and nuclear power industry have made extensive use of simulation for training. In these industries, as in medicine, on-the-job training requires assumption of high risk.

There are also examples of simulation in medical education throughout history. Models have long been used to help students learn about anatomic structures. In China in 1027 AD, the imperial physician Wang Wei-Yi had 2 life-size bronze statues made for teaching surface anatomy and location of acupuncture points.[15,16] In the eighteenth century, 2 surgeons working separately in Bologna and Paris developed birthing simulator models to teach delivery techniques to address high infant and maternal mortality rates.[13–15,17]

The movement toward the modern era of medical simulation began in the 1960s. At the beginning of the decade, a toy manufacturer named Ausmund Laerdal worked alongside anesthesiologists to design a simulator to teach mouth-to-mouth ventilation. The mannequin became known as Resusci-Anne and revolutionized resuscitation training by a low-cost, readily available, effective training model.[14,18,19] An internal spring was later attached to the mannequin's chest wall, permitting cardiac compression simulation. In 1968, Dr Michael Gordon presented Harvey, a cardiology patient simulator, to the American Heart Association.[14]

Around the same time that Resusci-Anne was introduced, another type of simulation was being developed. In 1964, Howard Barrows, a young academic neurologist, began to use actors to simulate neurologic signs and symptoms in lessons with his students.[14] Patient actors, more commonly termed "standardized patients" (SPs), are now the most widely used simulation mode in medical education. Significant technological improvements throughout the 1980s and 1990s allowed the development of software and computerized systems that could be added to educational scenarios to mimic physiologic responses and provide real-time feedback.

Most medical schools and residency programs have integrated formal simulation programs into their curricula. "Doctoring" courses routinely make use of SP interviews for both learning and assessment.[20,21] Standardized patient assessments are such an integral part of modern medical education assessment that the US Medical Licensing Examination Step 2 Clinical Skills Examination, the national standardized examination that assesses medical students' interview skills, physical examination aptitude, and professionalism, uses SPs for each encounter. Although SPs are one of the most commonly used types of simulation in medical education, there are a multitude of other simulation methods used today, from low-technology anatomic models to high-fidelity patient simulators.

EDUCATIONAL THEORY

SBME allows experiential learning to take place in a setting removed from the risks of patient care with easier opportunities for observation and feedback. Traditionally, the preclinical phase of medical school is devoted to didactic teaching, while the clinical years of medical school and most of residency are focused on experiential learning. Experiential learning is acknowledged as the cornerstone of medical education in that it "operates with the principle that experience imprints knowledge more readily than didactic or online presentations alone."[22]

Integrating simulation in the preclinical curriculum provides experiential learning sessions to complement classroom didactics. For residents and clinical-year students, simulation allows experiential learning to take place in a structured, standardized format. David Kolb described 4 stages in the experiential learning cycle: "concrete experience (an event), reflective observation (what happened), abstract conceptualization (what was learned, future implications), and active experimentation (what will be done differently)."[22] Compared with traditional on-the-job training, SBME better facilitates the second, third, and fourth stages. In the clinical setting, the constraints of patient care mean that there is limited time and mentorship for reflective observation and abstract conceptualization. In addition, active experimentation is easily accomplished in SBME because trainees can practice the same scenario repeatedly.

SIMULATION MODALITIES

See **Table 1** for the characteristics of the different modalities used in SBME.

USE OF SIMULATION-BASED MEDICAL EDUCATION IN PSYCHIATRY

Simulation is widely used in medical education, including in psychiatry. Approximately 45% of medical schools and 12% of teaching hospitals reported incorporating simulation in the psychiatry clerkship for medical students.[4] More than 20% of medical schools and 5% of teaching hospitals use simulation in psychiatry residency curriculum.

Although a late adopter of SBME, in recent years psychiatry has had "rapid growth in simulation implementation and innovation."[22] SP encounters are by far the most commonly used simulation type in psychiatric education,[32] although there is also published research on using screen-based computer simulation for psychiatry training and opportunities for exploring other simulation modalities.

Use of Standardized Patients

SPs are widely used for teaching interview skills to trainees. SP interviews are especially helpful for exposing students to a broader range of psychopathology than they might encounter in their clinical rotations alone and for simulating high-risk scenarios such as suicidal patients.[24] Common applications of SPs include helping students learn the content and structure of the mental status examination[22] and helping residents practice psychotherapy.[33,34]

Interactions with SPs are also used to assess trainee' competencies in psychiatry, ranging from the mental status examination to assessment of suicide risk.[35,36] Objective structured clinical examinations (OSCEs) are a common method for evaluating students' interview skills in the psychiatry clerkship.[24] Evaluation scores are based on both objective checklist items and subjective measurements of a trainee's interpersonal skills, which may be scored by faculty and/or SPs.[22] Two studies have shown that OSCE scores correlate well with other assessments of the trainees, such as preceptor evaluations on wards, which helps validate the use of OSCEs.[37,38] For both faculty and SP scores, reliability is increased with greater number and variety of OSCE stations,[39] with 6 to 10 observations per domain suggested for reliable assessment.[27]

As SPs are increasingly used in psychiatric education, some investigators have cautioned educators to be mindful of the limitations of SPs in teaching and assessing complex interpersonal skills. In psychiatry, SPs may find it especially difficult to portray pathology realistically. Certain complex skills required for psychiatry are inherently hard for trainees to practice in a fabricated encounter; these include teasing out delusions from deliberate lies and recognizing truths that the patient has not yet explicitly acknowledged.[24] Brenner[24] suggests that SPs are most effective in teaching and assessing "discrete skills," such as covering all components of the Mental Status Examination (MSE), rather than complex interpersonal skills like emotional responsiveness and empathy.

Table 1
Characteristics of different simulation modalities

Simulation Modalities and Description	Applicable Competencies	Limitations in Psychiatric Education	Resource Requirements
Low-technology models • Anatomic models • Inert mannequins	• Anatomic knowledge • Procedural skills	• Limited applications in psychiatry • Limited ability to respond to trainee input	• Lower start-up and maintenance costs • Instructor needed for any substantial feedback
Standardized patients • Actors or lay persons trained to portray patient scenarios	• Patient interview skills, including those involving complex conversation[22] • Physical examination skills • Professionalism • Crisis management[23]	• Limited ability to teach or assess complex interpersonal skills due to the explicit falseness of the scenario[24,25] • Difficulty simulating abnormal physical examination findings[26] • Variable reliability depending on experience, skill, and training of the SP[26] as well as case number, length, and order[27] • Demonstrated relationship between experience with SPs and performance on OSCEs, which suggests a "possible practice effect or test-taking behavior"[28]	• SP salaries • High administrative costs for recruiting and training the "SP bank"[26] • Significant faculty time required for writing cases, facilitating teaching sessions, and evaluating performance on OSCEs[29]
Screen-based computer simulation • Interactive computer programs that return different outputs based on trainee input[27]	• Patient interview skills • Clinical decision making • Crisis management	• Preprogrammed actions and responses; not adaptable[30] • Limited ability to teach and evaluate interpersonal skills[27]	• Expensive to develop or purchase[31] • Ongoing costs: equipment maintenance and software upgrades

(continued on next page)

Table 1
(continued)

Simulation Modalities and Description	Applicable Competencies	Limitations in Psychiatric Education	Resource Requirements
Complex task trainers • Anatomic or surgical models integrated with computer programs to provide high-fidelity procedural trainings	• Procedural skills	• Limited applications in psychiatry	• Expensive systems (>15K) • Ongoing costs: other equipment beyond that included with the model, equipment maintenance, and software upgrades
High-fidelity patient simulators • Mannequins integrated with computer systems, typically capable of simulating physical examination findings (eg, pulses and breathing sounds) and displaying other relevant information (eg, patient demographics, laboratory results)	• Physical examination skills • Clinical decision making • Crisis management • Team work	• Not capable of complex conversations	• Extremely expensive systems (~250K)[27]
Virtual reality (VR) Interactive system with sensory input (eg, audiovisual, tactile) combined with user receptors (eg, head or body trackers)[5,30]	• Patient interview skills • Physical examination skills • Clinical decision making • Crisis management • Team work • Procedural skills	• Preprogrammed actions and responses; not adaptable[30] • Limited nonverbal communication cues[30] • Faculty evaluator required for assessing interpersonal skills	• Limited existing programs and templates • High start-up costs

Abbreviations: OSCE, objective structured clinical examination; SP, standardized patient.

Use of Screen-Based Computer Simulation

Computer simulations of the psychiatric interview were discussed in the literature as early as 1967,[40] but application has been limited. Beutler and Harwood[5] piloted a psychotherapy simulation with a 2-dimensional virtual patient displayed on a computer screen. As the trainee talked to the display, a trained observer categorized the trainee's questions or interventions and chose the appropriate preprogrammed response for the virtual patient, based on a branching logic. Another group developed a Web-based simulation that involved selecting actions from multiple choice lists to assess psychiatry residents' competency in obtaining informed consent for antipsychotics.[41] During pilot testing, residents reported that this simulation was easy to use and helped increase their confidence in obtaining informed consent.[42]

Computer simulations of psychiatric encounters, however, are limited in their ability to realistically portray complex social interactions. With current technology, each response must be preprogrammed and it is difficult to create scripts that are adaptable and detailed enough to simulate a psychiatric interview or a psychotherapy session. Artificial intelligence (AI) may eventually be used to simulate complex conversation,[5] but currently, that application is mostly speculative.

Telehealth training is a particularly promising application for virtual patients, because telehealth competency is becoming increasingly important for psychiatrists and telehealth encounters involve only audio or 2-dimensional displays.

Use of High-Fidelity Patient Simulators and Virtual Reality

Limited experience has been published for using high-fidelity patient simulators or virtual reality in psychiatric education. Virtual reality systems offer the unique opportunity to track trainee gaze direction and body positioning,[30] which could be useful for providing feedback on unconscious signaling during psychiatric interviews.

Other Applications for Simulation

Beyond teaching and assessment, simulation has been used to foster understanding and empathy for patients among trainees.[22] The most common application is using voice recordings, often based on patients' real hallucinations, to simulate auditory hallucinations for students.[22] Recently, Yellowlees and Cook[43] piloted an Internet-based virtual reality system to simulate the audio and visual hallucinations of a person with schizophrenia.

Financing for Simulation Programs

Few programs publish information on costs of individual simulations or simulation programs, and there are no published data on psychiatry-specific spending for educational simulation. In the AAMC survey on simulation programs, the annual operating budgets reported by medical schools were evenly split between the different budget categories (from \$0–250,000 to >\$1,000,000).[4] Respondents varied widely in the types of administrative costs they included.

Eighty-four percent of medical schools and 90% of teaching hospitals reported that they had complete or partial ownership over their simulation facilities. The most commonly reported funding sources were the medical school (87%), grants (40%), and courses and services to groups and individuals (33%).[4] The vast majority of medical schools and hospitals (90% overall) reported sharing the simulation facilities with other health professionals and even nonclinical entities, such as industry.[4]

Current Evidence on Outcomes and Benefits

Research has shown that using simulation in psychiatry education improves educational outcomes, including adherence to interview protocols and assessment scores.[44,45] Trainees report finding standardized patient activities in psychiatry education useful and satisfying.[46,47] Simulation, including Web-based experiences, can also help trainees and members of the general population understand and empathize with psychiatric symptoms.[43,48] However, evidence is limited for more distant impacts. For example, a recent systematic review identified 48 articles on outcomes of psychiatry-related SBME but none of the studies investigated patient outcomes.[44] Outside of psychiatry, studies have shown that SBME is associated with positive outcomes at multiple translational levels, including in patient care practices, patient outcomes, and collateral effects such as cost savings.[9]

CASE STUDY ON UNSTABLE PATIENT SIMULATION

Since 2009, all medical students at MUSC have participated in an unstable patient simulation on a high-fidelity patient simulator during their third-year psychiatry clerkship.[49] The simulation center at MUSC opened in June 2008, funded by donors for the purpose of improving patient safety. The center has 11,000 square feet with 14 simulation rooms.

The interactive mannequin used for the psychiatry simulation displays vital signs and case information on a computer screen and a resident or attending serves as the voice of the patient. In the simulation, the mannequin's parameters respond according to a branching algorithm based on the actions taken by the students in the simulated examination room. The actions are entered into the computer system by an instructor sitting in a control room adjacent to the simulated examination room. This instructor additionally speaks to the student team over the phone throughout the case. In total, 2 preceptors are needed for each simulation activity: one serving as the patient voice for the mannequin and the other acting as attending on call and recording the actions of the students. The team has developed pre-reading materials for students, teaching points for instructors for the debrief, and a suggested script for the patient actor.

The simulation involves 2 urgent management cases, one on alcohol withdrawal and delirium management and the other on neuroleptic malignant syndrome. In each session, there are 6 to 8 students split into 2 groups. Students complete one of the simulation cases and observe the other case. The cases lasted approximately 15 minutes each, with the timeline accelerated well beyond real-life scenarios. Immediately after the case, one of the preceptors led a debriefing session.

Throughout the 4 years of experience, the team has modified several elements of the simulation. Early on, students completed a post-activity quiz, but this was dropped because it was felt to add undue stress while returning minimal value. To improve teamwork and ensure individual participation, each student on the 4-person team is now assigned a specific role. Based on student feedback, the preceptors have been encouraged to offer more interjections during the case, such as confirming the medication dose the students want, and framed this expanded involvement as an "attending on call" role.

Over the past 4 years, students and preceptors have consistently given positive feedback on the simulation activity. This simulation adds value to the MUSC psychiatry clerkship as evidenced by the overwhelmingly positive ratings. Measuring the long-term impact on patient care has been challenging for many reasons, including inability to follow students' clinical experiences after their clerkship, student attrition to other institutions postgraduation, and low percentage of students pursuing psychiatry as a career choice.

RECOMMENDATIONS FOR INCORPORATING SIMULATION IN PSYCHIATRIC EDUCATION
Content and Competencies

In psychiatry, simulation is especially useful for teaching and assessing discrete interview skills such as completing the MSE and competencies related to unstable patient management. As other investigators have expounded,[24] at the present time simulation is not well suited to teaching and assessing complex interpersonal skills.

Appropriate resources should be devoted to researching, writing, and piloting simulation cases. We suggest developing pre-reading materials, patient and preceptor scripts, and teaching points, as appropriate for the purpose of the activity.

Educators should view simulation as an opportunity for interprofessional training. In health care settings, teams are usually composed of members from different fields, specialties, and training levels, yet training remains siloed. Preclinical trainees are typically segregated by discipline, and while clinical trainees work on interdisciplinary teams, it is rare for them to have integrated training or education sessions. Simulation offers an ideal opportunity to practice team work for high-risk scenarios. Simulation centers are an especially easy setting for collaborative training because they are often jointly funded by different schools and departments.

Simulation Modalities

SPs remain the preferred modality for any scenarios that require complex social interaction, because all other technologies are limited in their ability to simulate realistic conversation. Computer-based simulations are best suited for discrete interview skills and clinical decision-making algorithms. In the case of high-fidelity patient simulators like mannequins, scenarios with physiologic findings (eg, unstable vital signs, critical laboratory results) tend to use the technology more fully. Unstable patient situations will be best represented by SPs if they require complex conversations (eg, suicidal or homicidal patients) and by interactive mannequins or computer-based simulations if they involve more physiologic findings.

Virtual reality holds the potential to provide immersive simulated experiences and will be especially useful for competencies in clinical decision making and crisis management. Virtual reality systems also have already shown potential for fostering empathy for patients. Low-technology models and complex task trainers have limited role in psychiatry; they may be useful in teaching neuroanatomy and some aspects of interventional psychiatry procedures.

Simulation Activity Structure

We recommend including a debriefing session in all educational simulation activities. The debrief should be used to cover relevant learning points and to provide feedback. Debriefing facilitates the reflective observation stage of Kolb's experiential learning cycle[22] and is recognized as crucial for the effectiveness of simulation-based learning.[50]

For most simulations, immersion and believability will be improved by having minimal instructor interjections during the activity. In our experience, incorporating an "attending on call" role can minimize student frustration and prevent them from making egregious mistakes that would end the simulation scenario abruptly. Where time and equipment resources are limited, having trainees participate in the simulation in groups is a feasible option and has some benefits over individual participation, including minimizing trainee embarrassment, allowing for teamwork practice, and encouraging interprofessional collaboration.

Simulation Program Funding

Using SPs requires not just salaries for the SPs but also sufficient funds and infrastructure for recruiting, training, and preparing the SPs. Other simulation types may have higher upfront development costs and still have ongoing financing needs, including equipment maintenance and software upgrades. For all simulation types, there are administrative costs related to running the program, which should not be overlooked while developing the program. Mechanisms for long-term operating costs should be considered from the start of the program, especially if the initial funding came from a one-time source such as a donation or grant.

Sharing simulation facilities with other health professions may help secure and maintain adequate funding for the simulation programs. For example, 21% of medical schools that filled out the AAMC simulation survey reported that the nursing school contributed funding for simulation programs.[4]

DISCUSSION

In traditional medical training, it is hard to provide a gradual escalation of responsibility in the transitions from preclinical student to clinical student to resident to fully boarded physician. For airplane pilots, training often incorporates a "ride-along" instructor who can take control of the flight at any time. Medical training, especially in the field of psychiatry, does not allow for such close supervision or the ability for a supervisor to seamlessly assume control of the situation.

As described in the literature, SBME offers the chance for learners to take on greater degrees of responsibility in low-risk settings, provides time for reflection and feedback, and allows repetitive practice in the same scenario. When simulation activities are immersive and realistic, they facilitate substantial experiential learning. Simulation also allows for structured, standardized assessments. Because of these advantages, simulation has been hailed as a method for improving trainee competence and ultimately patient safety. Research shows positive impacts at multiple levels of translational outcomes for general SBME, though data are more limited in psychiatry education.

Going forward, we expect to see greater incorporation of computer-based simulation, high-fidelity patient simulators, and virtual reality simulations in SBME, especially as these technologies improve and become more accessible. AI may one day replace the branching logic used in most simulation methods so that the range of possible reactions and scenarios is not limited by what was preprogrammed. This could allow systems to respond fluidly to trainee input and realistically simulate conversation, which is currently a major deficiency in all simulations that do not involve SPs.

Simulation provides an ideal setting for practicing team dynamics, but currently there is little published experience on incorporating interprofessional teams in psychiatric simulations. We hope to see more research and reports on this topic in the near future.

In psychiatry, there has been limited research on how SBME programs impact more distant implementation outcomes, especially care practices and patient outcomes. Improving patient safety is a key goal of simulation programs and demonstrating evidence would help secure and justify funding for simulation programs.

CLINICS CARE POINTS

- SBME offers multiple advantages over traditional clinical training: there is no risk of patient harm during learning, scenarios are standardized, instructors can directly and discreetly observe trainees, there is time for feedback and debriefing, and trainees can practice the same scenario repetitively.

- SBME has been shown to improve outcomes at multiple translational levels. In psychiatry, research has demonstrated that SBME results in improved educational outcomes and reduced stigma around mental health disorders.

- In psychiatry, competencies recommended for SBME include discrete interview skills, unstable patient management, and team management. SBME is also an opportunity to expose students to a broader range of psychopathology than they are likely to encounter through clinical rotations.

- Simulation modalities include low-technology models (eg, anatomic models, inert mannequins), standardized patients, screen-based computer simulations, complex task trainers, high-fidelity patient simulators (eg, interactive mannequins), and virtual reality systems.

- Selecting a modality depends on educational goals and available resources. Certain scenarios are best portrayed by specific modalities, such as complex social interactions by standardized patients and unstable vital signs by high-fidelity patient simulators

- Simulation programs are expensive to initiate and maintain. Sharing costs between multiple departments and institutions will help to alleviate the financing burden and additionally may serve as an impetus for increased interprofessional SMBE training.

DISCLOSURE

The authors have nothing to disclose.

REFERENCES

1. McGaghie WC. Mastery learning: it is time for medical education to join the 21st century. Acad Med 2015;90(11):1438–41.
2. Kohn LT, Corrigan JM, Donaldson MS, editors. To err is human: building a safer health system. Washington DC: National Academics Press; 2000.
3. Armenia S, Thangamathesvaran L, Caine AD, et al. The role of high-fidelity team-based simulation in acute care settings: a systematic review. Surg J 2018;4(03): e136–51.
4. Passiment M, Sacks H, Huang G. Medical simulation in medical education: results of an AAMC survey. Washington, DC: Association of American Medical Colleges; 2011.
5. Beutler LE, Harwood TM. Virtual reality in psychotherapy training. J Clin Psychol 2004;60(3):317–30.
6. Ziv A, Small SD, Wolpe PR. Patient safety and simulation-based medical education. Med Teach 2000;22(5):489–95.
7. Ziv A, Wolpe PR, Small SD, et al. Simulation-based medical education: an ethical imperative. Acad Med 2003;78(8):783–8.
8. Cook DA, Brydges R, Zendejas B, et al. Mastery learning for health professionals using technology-enhanced simulation: a systematic review and meta-analysis. Acad Med 2013;88(8):1178–86.
9. McGaghie WC, Issenberg SB, Barsuk JH, et al. A critical review of simulation-based mastery learning with translational outcomes. Med Educ 2014;48(4): 375–85.
10. Sperling JD, Clark S, Kang Y. Teaching medical students a clinical approach to altered mental status: simulation enhances traditional curriculum. Med Educ Online 2013;18(1):19775.

11. Lentz GM, Mandel LS, Goff BA. A six-year study of surgical teaching and skills evaluation for obstetric/gynecologic residents in porcine and inanimate surgical models. Am J Obstet Gynecol 2005;193(6):2056–61.
12. Jónasson JT. Educational change, inertia and potential futures. Eur J Futures Res 2016;4(1):7.
13. Rosen KR. The history of medical simulation. J Crit Care 2008;23(2):157–66.
14. Jones F, Passos-Neto CE, Braghiroli OFM. Simulation in medical education: brief history and methodology. Principles Pract Clin Res 2015;1(2).
15. Owen H. Early use of simulation in medical education. Simul Healthc 2012;7(2): 102–16.
16. Schnorrenberger CC. Anatomical roots of Chinese medicine and acupuncture. Schweiz Z Fur Ganzheitsmed 2008;20(3):163.
17. Buck GH. Development of simulators in medical education. Gesnerus 1991;48 Pt 1:7–28.
18. Bradley P. The history of simulation in medical education and possible future directions. Med Educ 2006;40(3):254–62.
19. Cooper J, Taqueti V. A brief history of the development of mannequin simulators for clinical education and training. Postgrad Med J 2008;84(997):563–70.
20. Hawkins S, Osborne A, Schofield SJ, et al. Improving the accuracy of self-assessment of practical clinical skills using video feedback–the importance of including benchmarks. Med Teach 2012;34(4):279–84.
21. Wang EE. Simulation and adult learning. Dis Mon 2011;57(11):664–78.
22. Levine AI, DeMaria S, Schwartz AD, et al. The comprehensive textbook of healthcare simulation. New York: Springer Science & Business Media; 2013.
23. Hall MJ, Adamo G, McCurry L, et al. Use of standardized patients to enhance a psychiatry clerkship. Acad Med 2004;79(1):28–31.
24. Brenner AM. Uses and limitations of simulated patients in psychiatric education. Acad Psychiatry 2009;33(2):112–9.
25. Krahn LE, Bostwick JM, Sutor B, et al. The challenge of empathy: a pilot study of the use of standardized patients to teach introductory psychopathology to medical students. Acad Psychiatry 2002;26(1):26–30.
26. Cleland JA, Abe K, Rethans J-J. The use of simulated patients in medical education: AMEE Guide No 42. Med Teach 2009;31(6):477–86.
27. Srinivasan M, Wang JC, West D, et al. Assessment of clinical skills using simulator technologies. Acad Psychiatry 2006;30(6):505–15.
28. Talente G, Haist SA, Wilson JF. The relationship between experience with standardized patient examinations and subsequent standardized patient examination performance: a potential problem with standardized patient exam validity. Eval Health Prof 2007;30(1):64–74.
29. Patrício MF, Julião M, Fareleira F, et al. Is the OSCE a feasible tool to assess competencies in undergraduate medical education? Med Teach 2013;35(6):503–14.
30. Stevens A, Hernandez J, Johnsen K, et al. The use of virtual patients to teach medical students history taking and communication skills. Am J Surg 2006; 191(6):806–11.
31. Williams K, Wryobeck J, Edinger W, et al. Assessment of competencies by use of virtual patient technology. Acad Psychiatry 2011;35(5):328–30.
32. Abpool PS, Nirula L, Bonato S, et al. Simulation in undergraduate psychiatry: exploring the depth of learner engagement. Acad Psychiatry 2016;41(2):251–61.
33. Coyle B, Miller M, McGowen K. Using standardized patients to teach and learn psychotherapy. Acad Med 1998;73(5):591–2.

34. Klamen DL, Yudkowsky R. Using standardized patients for formative feedback in an introduction to psychotherapy course. Acad Psychiatry 2002;26(3):168–72.
35. Hodges BD, Hollenberg E, McNaughton N, et al. The psychiatry OSCE: a 20-year retrospective. Acad Psychiatry 2014;38(1):26–34.
36. Hung EK, Binder RL, Fordwood SR, et al. A method for evaluating competency in assessment and management of suicide risk. Acad Psychiatry 2012;36(1):23–8.
37. McLay RN, Rodenhauser P, Anderson DS, et al. Simulating a full-length psychiatric interview with a complex patient: an OSCE for medical students. Acad Psychiatry 2002;26(3):162–7.
38. Whelan P, Church L, Kadry K. Using standardized patients' marks in scoring postgraduate psychiatry OSCEs. Acad Psychiatry 2009;33(4):319–22.
39. Swanson DB, van der Vleuten CPM. Assessment of clinical skills with standardized patients: state of the art revisited. Teach Learn Med 2013;25(sup1):S17–25.
40. Starkweather JA, Kamp M, Monto A. Psychiatric interview simulation by computer. Methods Inf Med 1967;6(1):15–23.
41. Gorrindo T, Baer L, Sanders KM, et al. Web-based simulation in psychiatry residency training: a pilot study. Acad Psychiatry 2011;35(4):232–7.
42. Gorrindo T, Baer L, Sanders KM, Birnbaum RJ, Fromson JA, Sutton-Skinner KM, Romeo SA, Beresin EV. Web-based simulation in psychiatry residency training: a pilot study. Acad Psychiatry. 2011 Jul-Aug;35(4):232-237.
43. Yellowlees PM, Cook JN. Education about hallucinations using an internet virtual reality system: a qualitative survey. Acad Psychiatry 2006;30(6):534–9.
44. Williams B, Reddy P, Marshall S, et al. Simulation and mental health outcomes: a scoping review. Adv Simulation 2017;2(1):2.
45. Hayes-Roth B, Saker R, Amano K, et al. Automating individualized coaching and authentic role-play practice for brief intervention training. Methods Inf Med 2010; 49(04):406–11.
46. Hall M, Adamo G, McCurry L, et al. Use of standardized patients to enhance a psychiatric clerkship. Acad Med 2004;79(1):28–31.
47. Brown R, Doonan S, Shellenberger S, et al. Using children as simulated patients in communication training for residents and medical students: a pilot program. Acad Med 2005;80(12):1114–20.
48. Ballon BC, Silver I, Fidler D. Headspace theater: an innovative method for experiential learning of psychiatric symptomatology using modified role-playing and improvisational theater techniques. Acad Psychiatry 2007;31(5):380–7.
49. Funk M, Pelic CM, Pelic CG, et al. Simulation centers in consultation-liaison psychiatry education: a practical workshop. In: Academy of psychosomatic medicine 2015 annual meeting. 2015. New Orleans, LA.
50. Issenberg BS, McGaghie WC, Petrusa ER, et al. Features and uses of high-fidelity medical simulations that lead to effective learning: a BEME systematic review. Med Teach 2005;27(1):10–28.

Psychiatric Clinics
Computer-Based Teaching

John Luo, MD

KEYWORDS

- Distance learning • Computerized teaching • Computer-based teaching
- Technology for teaching

KEY POINTS

- Technology has become easier to use, much like the smartphone.
- A variety of tools are available to the medical educator to facilitate learning.
- Spend the time to learn advantages and disadvantages and adapt material to the tool.
- Use the key features of the tool to emphasize teaching points.

INTRODUCTION

Many US-based medical schools record their lectures as an accommodation for students with learning disabilities. Nowadays, many students take advantage of that resource and often do not bother coming to class. They will only attend a lecture when it is mandated for a guest speaker, such as a patient, who has generously taken time out of their schedule to share their experience with an illness. Students even prefer to watch the recorded lecture video from a lecture at double speed to get through the material quickly. They can watch these videos at the library, coffee shop, or wherever their preferred learning habitat is located. Students will even watch recorded lecture videos in the lecture hall on their laptop when attendance is mandated during another lecture! This example is just one of many ways that computers and technology have impacted the educational process.

Even though faculty often decry the loss of the time-honored tradition of the in-person lecture, it is no longer appropriate to "blame" the millennial generation for demanding that their teachers adapt to their preferred learning style. In fact, teaching using computer technology has been in place since the early 1970s.[1] Although much has changed over the years with both computer hardware and software, computer-based educational methods in medical education have been slowly adopted. The most popular use of computer-based education namely has been using presentation software, such as Microsoft PowerPoint, Apple Keynote, and Prezi. Presentation

UCI Health System, 101 The City Drive South, Orange, CA 92868, USA
E-mail address: johnluo@hs.uci.edu
Twitter: @jsluo (J.L.)

Psychiatr Clin N Am 44 (2021) 173–181
https://doi.org/10.1016/j.psc.2021.03.003
0193-953X/21/© 2021 Elsevier Inc. All rights reserved.

software has largely replaced the now archaic overhead and slide projectors, but few medical educators have ventured into adoption of newer technologies that emphasize engagement and active learning. This article reviews many of these computer-based teaching tools with the goal to stimulate their use even for those educators who think that they are not computer experts.

COMPUTER-BASED TEACHING TOOLS

One of the basic but effective ways to create an educational module online is to record a narration with Microsoft PowerPoint.[2] This feature is accessed under the "slide show" menu by selecting the option "record slide show." Audio narrations can be saved either for each slide or for the entire presentation. For the audio to add an extra element to the presentation, the key is to not merely read the words on the slide. Presentations should be created using style guides, such as those described on Presentation Zen.[3] An effective combination is to use a picture that captures a part of the story to be told, and therefore, the narration is key to the teaching points. There should be a clear theme to the slides, and the number of slides should be condensed to an essential number. When style creativity is a challenge, templates such as those available on Visme may help deliver the message.[4] The style theme often facilitates delivery of the message with both visuals and more intriguing layouts compared with the defaults in presentation software.

With recorded presentations, too long of a presentation will often lose the attention of the viewer. As a guideline, check out some of the videos posted on YouTube. Many of the videos with high view count tend to be between 12 and 15 minutes long. Of course, interesting content lends itself to being fully viewed; however, even the most diligent of students will need to break up content that is too long. The advantage of a narrated presentation is that it engages the reader beyond the outline of material typically seen in a presentation. Once the slideshow has been recorded, it can be hosted on a Web site, learning management system (LMS), wiki, blog, podcasting service, or just in cloud-based storage, such as DropBox. To further enhance learning, especially in a nonlinear manner, PowerPoint and Keynote both offer the ability to hyperlink slides for navigation with a click on an image or navigation icon. A good example of this type of presentation is a Jeopardy-style template, which is readily available on the Internet for download and use. This type of interactive presentation is ideal for individualized review of material but can also be used in an in-person class setting with the faculty member channeling their inner Alex Trebek.

Another software tool to consider is a screen-recording and video-editing software program, such as Camtasia.[5] In addition to recording the audio, Camtasia facilitates recording video via the Web cam on the desktop or laptop computer. It can integrate a recording toolbar directly into PowerPoint, thereby making it easier to start and stop a recording.[6] Although Camtasia is geared toward an individual license, many educational institutions use enterprise-level software, such as Panopto.[7] This software offers more features, such as integration with learning management platforms, such as Blackboard, Canvas, Moodle, and Sakai; search and index the video to capture keywords; create optimized videos for any device, such as smartphones; integrate video quizzes; and schedule recordings. Yuja is another enterprise-level video platform to consider.[8] It also manages video capture, integrates into many learning management platforms, provides a cloud platform for storage and streaming and in video quizzes, but also offers video examination proctoring tools as well as automated tools for accessibility, such as closed captioning, text-to-speech audio, and electronic braille.

Podcasts can also be an effective way to deliver educational content. These podcasts are primarily audio but can be video files that are downloaded to a listening device, such as a smartphone or computer, to be reviewed asynchronously when convenient. The key feature of a podcast is that it is typically a series of podcasts from the same hosts, and the learner can subscribe to receive automatic downloads when they become available. There are many guides to starting a podcast, such as the one from Podcast Insights.[9] A good-quality microphone, video camera, and editing software, such as Audacity, will be needed.[10] If editing, creating cover art, or adding background music and video are too much to handle, services, such as Alitu[11] and Resonate Recordings,[12] can address these issues so that educators can focus on content. Most successful podcasts are interview shows with guests because the topic and dialogue between the hosts and guests are more engaging. Podcasts can be hosted on a service, such as Buzzsprout, which can provide metrics, such as number of downloads, what apps people are using to listen to the podcast, and where they are listening.[13] Podcasts on Buzzsprout can be listed in Apple Podcasts, Spotify, Google Podcasts, Stitcher, iHeart Radio, TuneIn, Alexa, and many other services.

Presentation videos and podcasts can be hosted on popular sites, such as YouTube.[14] YouTube is considered the second most popular Web site in the world; therefore, presentations posted there can reach a very broad audience. Patients often post a video log or vlog about their experiences with mental illness, and many psychiatric clinics and hospitals are posting educational videos to help educate the public as well as use the brand awareness for marketing. One of the disadvantages is that their proprietary algorithm determines what other videos are recommended for viewers, not to mention that there is also no control what advertisements that Google will choose to display. For those reasons, organizations, such as the American Psychiatric Association, that need hosting services for their videos often choose other vendors, such as Vimeo.[15] Vimeo will provide analytics, such as number of views, what device was used, where the request came from, and which region the video was viewed in. More importantly, Vimeo provides full management of the video without ads, viewer limits, or overages. Vimeo also has tools, such as audience chat, live polls, live question and answer, and e-mail capture, that are part of their live streaming service.

Prezi is a different type of presentation software, which has unique features, such as zooming in on a picture to highlight a specific message.[16] By design, Prezi is already nonlinear and more visually based, which helps it be more engaging because of visual stimulation. For example, imagine seeing a picture of the brain, but instead of showing a next slide, the presentation zooms into a region where now the sulci and areas are labeled. The next step could be a shift to images and text describing symptoms of diseases with deficits from those locations. There is also a Prezi Video program that creates videos with the ability to add graphics and images as well as import PowerPoint. Prezi Designer creates infographics, posters, social media posts, and reports. A variety of templates help provide a starting point to craft the educational lesson with built-in graphics and charts. Although the initial learning curve can be challenging with developing Prezi presentations, videos, and designs, the large number of existing templates should minimize frustration. The main challenge of Prezi use is creativity in designing a potentially nonlinear learning experience using many of its features.

Interaction, especially with in-person lectures, is a key element for audience engagement. Presentation software can be also augmented with real-time polls. For example, Poll Everywhere is an online audience response system that creates multiple choice questions, word clouds, and question and answer problems for active participation.[17] Specialized hardware is not necessary because participants can use a computer, use a smartphone app, or text their response. This real-time engagement can be useful to the presenter to modify his pace or level of detail based on the choices made by the audience. Integration with PowerPoint or Keynote is managed with a downloaded software application. A similar product is Mentimeter, which works completely online.[18] Besides standard slide templates with bullet points and other formats, it has popular question types, such as ranking, word cloud, multiple choice, as well as question and answer, in addition to quizzes and ranking slides. Poll Everywhere has a few more features, but the add-in element sometimes may be difficult to get to work properly, whereas the simplicity of Mentimeter may be enough for most educators to use because it is one overall package. Both Poll Everywhere and Mentimeter are dependent upon access to the Internet via either wifi or cellular data to function, so their use will be impossible in classrooms and conference centers where Internet access is not available. Adobe Captivate can convert an existing PowerPoint presentation into a video and then add interactive features, such as knowledge check questions, as overlays on top of the presentation video.[19]

In a similar vein, Kahoot takes interaction to another level in the form of a competitive game.[20] Participants join via either computer or smartphone on a Web browser using the Kahoot game code, registering their participation by selecting a name, and then waiting to answer questions. Creating a Kahoot is easy because the questions allow only a choice of up to 4 answers, which are linked to a color and shape presented on the smartphone screen of the participants instead of numbers or letters. Videos and images can be put on the question screen with that help cue the answer or to just provide a background. The question may have only 1 answer or allow many answers to be correct, and the amount of time for questions to be answered can be set. Game participants are provided points based on speed to the correct answer. After each question is answered, a running tally of the highest scorers is shown. Much of the fun using Kahoot comes with the funky carnival-type music that the system will play while waiting for responses in addition to seeing who will win. A Kahoot question can ask for knowledge about a fact or simply be a survey question. Use of Kahoot has been most effective as a prelecture and postlecture game. The game before the lecture cues the learner as to what material will be covered in lecture, and the postlecture game tests what the learner has learned in the lecture. Overall, despite its campy music and whimsical font, Kahoot is an effective way to engage learners from elementary to higher education.

With the power of technology today, computer-based simulation with virtual reality is poised to potentially transform medical education. It had its humble beginnings with the Virtual Human Project, a publicly available 3-dimensional representation of the human body.[21] These MRI and computed tomographic slices have been downloaded, and then software incorporates these images into visualization tools, such as the VH Dissector for Medical Education.[22] When the virtual reality platform Second Life started in 2003, it was heralded as more than just a game. It was touted as the next major platform for education, business, and government. Government and business had to purchase "land" in Second Life in order to build their virtual office or town hall. Dr Peter Yellowlees, a psychiatrist at UC Davis Medical Center in Sacramento, California, created a Second Life virtual hallucination simulation so that people could experience auditory and visual hallucinations.[23] Children's Hospital Los Angeles is using virtual reality simulators to train resident physicians on how to manage emergencies, such as a life-threatening allergic reaction in a toddler.[24] In this simulator, the trainee wears a headset and interacts with the environment to learn the impact of the decisions they make, which prepares them for when these incidences happen in real life. Osso VR is a virtual reality surgical training and assessment platform that helps surgeons learn new procedures.[25] It uses cutaneous haptics technology to provide surgeons with a real feel of instruments as they manipulate them in surgery. In psychiatry, virtual reality would be a great training space to teach deescalation much as police officers do in a training simulator.[26]

Augmented reality is also another venue for computer-based training. In augmented reality, computer-generated images are superimposed on real-life structures much like the videogame Pokémon Go puts monsters in real world locations. At UCI Medical Center, augmented reality is used to train medical students and emergency medicine residents. A hologram of a patient is superimposed on a manikin to create a more life-like and responsive scenario.[24] Recently, UCI Emergency Medicine trainers used Google Glass in an augmented reality training for mass casualty incidents for health care providers, such as emergency medical technicians, paramedics, nurses, and physicians, in Saudi Arabia.[27] The study demonstrated that augmented reality training could be successfully delivered at an off-site location. The advantage of augmented reality is that a specialized virtual reality or Google Glass headset is not needed. 8thWall[28] and Ubiquity6[29] are platforms to help develop augmented reality experiences on a smartphone browser.

Medical students and resident physicians nowadays use question banks to test their knowledge. There are several online question authoring systems, such as Testshop[30] and Jamison.[31] Many LMS offer quizzes, such as Moodle[32] and Canvas.[33] Learning management systems offer far more than just quizzes and delivery of presentations. They help track outcomes, help manage assets, such as videos and presentations discussed earlier, and have built-in eLearning authoring tools. Students and faculty can share ideas in forums, submit assignments, and track grades. Many medical schools have invested in an LMS to link outcomes for accreditation site visits and reporting. Curriculum management platforms, such as Ilios,[34] are Web-based applications that collect, manage, analyze, and deliver curricular information. They identify what is being taught in courses and identify gaps and redundancies. Competencies can be mapped that for reporting attestations and accreditation. LMS, curriculum management, examination assessment platforms, and other educational software products often require an enterprise level commitment of the school, which includes information technology department support because of the level of integration that many of these systems need. Most faculty will often find that an existing system or several systems are already in place, and they should take advantage of that system because of the support and experience already in place. Expense is also an issue, and few professors have the technical know-how to install and program a free open source LMS, such as Moodle, along with a Web server, database, and the PHP scripting language.[35]

Some organizations have a dedicated group or initiative focused on educational technologies. University of California, Irvine, School of Medicine iMedED initiative started in 2010 to foster individualized and small-group learning.[36] In their digital transformation program, first-year medical students have an iPad that is loaded with their entire first-year curriculum, including outlines, handouts, and digital textbooks. Many medical applications are loaded onto the iPad, including applications to take notes and to record. Students also use a digital stethoscope, such as the EKO Core Digital Stethoscope, which captures ECG tracings and heart sounds.[37] IMedED has created a specific ultrasound iPad application to consult video tutorials while they perform bedside ultrasounds. There are thousands of applications for tablets and smartphones geared toward medical education, such as Visible Body, which has 3-dimensional models and dissections of anatomy to facilitate learning on the go.[38] University of Southern California has an Institute for Creative Technologies with leaders in artificial intelligence, virtual reality, graphics, and narrative communities to advance technologies to solve problems facing service members, students, and society.[39] It is well known for using video game engines to create a treatment platform for military servicemen with posttraumatic stress disorder and has many other research projects, such as sexual harassment and assault prevention and counterterrorism prepared- ness. The PAL3 (Personal Assistant for Life Long Learning) project is a prototype plat- form for delivering engaging and accessible education on mobile devices.[40] One of the hallmarks is an interactive agent "Pal" to engage and motivate learners using amusing animations and dialogue with students through natural language processing of voice and text. Faculty members fortunate enough to have such a resource on their campus, which may even be in the school of engineering or education, should take advantage and collaborate with these researchers with a technical background.

Distance learning via video conference traditionally has been a bridge to bring geographically distant learners together, and with the recent COVID-19 pandemic, it has come to the forefront as one of the most heavily used platforms for teaching. The ability to deliver lectures in person while permitting social distancing and removing the barrier of travel has made mastery of this technology invaluable. Many medical schools and residency training programs during the pandemic moved their lectures immediately to video conferencing, and many conferences have done so as well. There are many advantages and disadvantages with the multitude of vendors, such as Zoom,[41] BlueJeans,[42] and GoToMeeting,[43] to name a few. In general, the free version will have limits, such as meeting length or number of participants. Most med- ical schools or hospital systems have an enterprise license for a specific vendor, which may dictate one's choice. Whichever system is used, educators should learn its fea- tures, such as the ability to secure the video conference with a security code, share a screen, use annotations, mute participants, and discuss how to expel an unwelcome participant. In addition, learning how to run an effective virtual meeting is also a must, such as being a good facilitator and setting ground rules.[44]

Over the years, social media has crossed from purely personal use into a blend of personal and professional use. Nowadays, medical educators can meet online, such as the @MedEdChat on Twitter, which meets on Thursday nights at 9 PM Eastern Standard Time.[45] Discussion topics are whatever is on the minds of participants, such as integrating telemedicine into training and how to optimize the physical learning environment for teaching. In the world of Twitter, hashtags #meded and #mededchat will help find interesting posts regarding medical education. Facebook also hosts many groups, whether it is on medical education, medical educators, or educational technology. In a quick look at the Facebook group on Education Technology,[46] Lisa Hegarty shared a link on Google Tools for Education. This link is a remote learning resource made available by Aquila Education, on how to create Google Forms for attendance or how to setup appointment slots with Google Calendar and Meet.[47] You- Tube is also a source of educational instruction on how to use Google forms as well as Calendar and Meet, but there is a sea of videos to review to find the most useful one.

SUMMARY

Computer-based teaching comes in many different forms of technology, ranging from hardware to software as well as from intuitive to requiring extensive training and sup- port. Although it is impossible to always please the learners, educators need to adapt to new technologies to enhance educational effectiveness. Few professors want their teaching to be considered passé by their audience because the technology they use or the educational content has not changed in 10 years. Adult learners benefit in comprehension and retention of material when they interact with both the teacher and the content.[48] For the millennial learner, understanding their attitudes, ideas, and priorities to tailor educational methods to stimulate and enhance learning is necessary for medical educators to customize their curricula and teaching methods to maximize learning.[49] Even social media is no longer considered too avant-garde or controversial in medical education.[50] The millennial learner enjoys collaborative learning, performs well in groups, and is technologically savvy.[51] Therefore, as educators, it is imperative to spend the time and energy to learn how to incorporate these new technologies in the classroom, online, and at conferences. If the approach is novel and would help other educators, it may benefit the faculty as a scholarly activity in a publication such as the MedEdPORTAL.[52]

CLINICS CARE POINTS

- Academic psychiatrists need to adjust their teaching style and the technology used to deliver educational content to reach today's learners. Learning to use new computer-based tools will help them engage the audience.
- In converting a lecture into a video, educators need to adapt the lecture with visually engaging content, interactive features, and appropriate length. Learning how to best use computer-based tools is essential to be an effective educator.
- Interactivity is a key element for audience engagement, implementing embedded videos, polls, quizzes, and games to keep the audience in active learning.
- Learning via videoconferencing software has become an important tool for distance learning and in the COVID-19 pandemic. Mastering use of the platform is essential to making the experience effective.
- Social media has become an important professional medium for discussing and distributing educational content, with hashtags and likes becoming as important as the number of times an article has been referenced.

DISCLOSURE

The author has nothing to disclose.

REFERENCES

1. Trzebiatowski GL, Ferguson IC. Computer technology in medical education. Med Prog Technol 1973;1(4):178–86.
2. Record presentations. Available at: https://support.office.com/en-us/article/video-record-presentations-2570dff5-f81c-40bc-b404-e04e95ffab33. Accessed April 3, 2020.
3. Reynolds G. 10 tips for improving your presentations today. Available at: https://www.presentationzen.com/. Accessed April 3, 2020.
4. Visme. Available at: https://www.visme.co/. Accessed April 20, 2020.
5. Camtasia. Available at: https://www.techsmith.com/video-editor.html. Accessed April 4, 2020.
6. Camtasia PowerPoint add-in toolbar. Available at: https://www.techsmith.com/tutorial-camtasia-ppt-addin-toolbar.html. Accessed April 4, 2020.
7. Panopto for education. Available at: https://www.panopto.com/panopto-for-education/. Accessed April 4, 2020.
8. Yuja. Available at: https://www.yuja.com/. Accessed April 5, 2020.

9. Winn R. How to start a podcast: a complete step-by-step tutorial. Available at: https://www.podcastinsights.com/start-a-podcast/. Accessed April 15, 2020.

10. Audacity. Available at: https://www.audacityteam.org/. Accessed April 15, 2020.

11. Alitu. Available at: https://alitu.com/. Accessed April 15, 2020.

12. Resonate recordings. Available at: https://resonaterecordings.com/. Accesed April 15, 2020.

13. Buzzsprout. Available at: https://www.buzzsprout.com/. Accessed April 15, 2020.

14. YouTube. Available at: https://www.youtube.com/. Accessed April 16, 2020.

15. Vimeo. Available at: https://vimeo.com/. Accessed April 16, 2020.

16. Prezi. Available at: https://prezi.com/. Accessed April 5, 2020.

17. Poll everywhere. Available at: https://www.polleverywhere.com/. Accessed April 5, 2020.

18. Mentimeter. Available at: https://www.mentimeter.com/. Accessed April 6, 2020.

19. Adobe captivate. Available at: https://www.adobe.com/products/captivate.html. Accessed April 15, 2020.

20. Kahoot. Available at: https://create.kahoot.it/. Accessed April 6, 2020.

21. Virtual Human Project. Available at: https://www.nlm.nih.gov/research/visible/visible_human.html. Accessed April 20, 2020.

22. VH Dissector for Medical Education. Available at: https://www.toltech.net/anatomy-software/solutions/vh-dissector-for-medical-education. Accessed April 20, 2020.

23. Yellowlees P. Virtual hallucinations. Available at: https://www.youtube.com/watch?v=s33Y5nl5Wbc. Accessed April 30, 2020.

24. Breining G. Future or fad? Virtual reality in medical education. Available at: https://www.aamc.org/news-insights/future-or-fad-virtual-reality-medical-education. Accessed April 30, 2020.

25. Osso VR. Available at: https://ossovr.com/. Accessed April 30, 2020.

26. Deescalation training for police officers. Available at: https://www.apexofficer.com/deescalation-training. Accessed April 30, 2020.

27. McCoy CE, Alrabah R, Weichmann W, et al. Feasibility of telesimulation and Google glass for mass casualty triage education and training. West J Emerg Med 2019;20(3):512–9.

28. 8thWall. Available at: https://www.8thwall.com/. Accessed April 30, 2020.

29. Ubiquity6. Available at: https://ubiquity6.com/#intro. Accessed April 30, 2020.

30. Testshop. Available at: https://www.testshop.com/desktop-network-internet-test-making-and-delivery. Accessed April 30, 2020.

31. Janison. Available at: https://www.janison.com/. Accessed April 30, 2020.

32. Moodle Plugin Studentquiz. Available at: https://moodle.org/plugins/. Accessed April 30, 2020.

33. Canvas quizzes. Available at: https://community.canvaslms.com/docs/DOC-10706. Accessed April 30, 2020.

34. Ilios. Available at: https://www.iliosproject.org/about/. Accessed April 30, 2020.

35. Moodle downloads. Available at: https://download.moodle.org. Accessed April 30, 2020.

36. IMedED initiative. Available at: http://www.meded.uci.edu/educational-technology/imeded-about.asp. Accessed April 30, 2020.

37. Eko CORE digital stethoscope. Available at: https://www.ekohealth.com. Accessed April 30, 2020.

38. Visible body. Available at: https://www.visiblebody.com/en-us/. Accessed April 30, 2020.

39. USC institute for creative technologies. Available at: https://ict.usc.edu/about/. Accessed April 30, 2020.
40. Personal Assistant for Life Long Learning. Available at: https://ict.usc.edu/prototypes/personal-assistant-for-life-long-learning-pal3/. Accessed April 30, 2020.
41. Zoom. Available at: https://www.zoom.us. Accessed April 30, 2020.
42. BlueJeans. Available at: https://www.bluejeans.com. Accessed April 30, 2020.
43. GoToMeeting. Available at: https://www.gotomeeting.com. Accessed April 30, 2020.
44. How to run effective virtual meetings. Available at: https://www.mindtoolscom/pages/article/running-effective-virtual-meetings.htm. Accessed April 30, 2020.
45. MedEd Chat. Available at: https://www.twitter.com/MedEdChat/. Accessed May 1, 2020.
46. Education technology. Available at: https://www.facebook.com/groups/379514775404784/. Accessed May 1, 2020.
47. Remote learning resources. Available at: https://www.aquilaeducation.com/remotelearning. Accessed May 1, 2020.
48. Chapman T. Waking up your lecture. Pediatr Radiol 2018;48:1388–92. https://doi.org/10.1007/s00247-018-4199-4.
49. Hopkins L, Hampton BS, Abbott JF, et al. To the point: medical education, technology, and the millennial learner. Am J Obstet Gynecol 2018;218(2):188–92.
50. Hillman T, Sherbino J. Social media in medical education: a new pedagogical paradigm? Postgrad Med J 2015;91(1080):544 5.
51. Schwartz AC, McDonald WM, Vahabzadeh AB, et al. Keeping up with changing times in education: fostering lifelong learning of millennial learners. Focus (Am Psychiatr Publ) 2018;16(1):74–9.
52. MedEdPORTAL. Available at: https://www.mededportal.org/. Accessed May 1, 2020.

Creating Successful Presentations

Carlyle H. Chan, MD

KEYWORDS

- Lectures • Death by PowerPoint • Presentation software • Lecture style

KEY POINTS

- Reflect on learning, audience, and content before constructing your presentation.
- Make slides that augment rather than distract from your presentation.
- Focus on one idea per slide, minimizing words and bullet points.
- Practice different aspects of your delivery that will help you engage your audience.

INTRODUCTION

In recent years, educators have promoted alternative methods of teaching, such as problem-based learning, flipped classrooms, case-based learning, and more. None have totally replaced the lecture format, particularly for conveying information to large groups of people. Nevertheless, lectures also continue to receive their share of criticism, as they may not be suitable for higher-order levels of thinking (eg, synthesis and analysis), are often data dumps of information, and may be offered by less than effective speakers.[1] Too often lectures are a passive learning exercise that fails to engage learners. A lecture goal is to create a more entertaining and active learning process that promotes learning and retention of the information being conveyed.

DISCUSSION

A successful presentation requires the application of 3 elements. These elements are reflection, augmentation, and delivery.

Reflection

In preparation for a lecture, the speaker needs to use reflection that entails contemplation, planning, and preparation. Initial attention should focus on what you want your listeners to learn and how they learn. There are many other considerations as well. For example, ask yourself these questions: Who is your intended audience, and what is their level of knowledge? You may need to pitch your talk differently when

Department of Psychiatry & Behavioral Medicine, Medical College of Wisconsin, 8701 Watertown Plank Road, Milwaukee, WI 53226, USA
E-mail address: cchan@mcw.edu

Psychiatr Clin N Am 44 (2021) 183–196
https://doi.org/10.1016/j.psc.2021.03.004
0193-953X/21/© 2021 Elsevier Inc. All rights reserved.

speaking to medical students versus colleagues versus the lay public. Consider the important points you wish to emphasize and how will you sequence your presentation. Ask yourself how you might enhance the learning of your audience? Will you need to prepare slides? Will you even need slides?

When we look for a model presentation, consider Abraham Lincoln's *Gettysburg Address*. This speech was one of history's most memorable. It consisted of 278 words and was delivered without visual aids. One of your key decisions is whether you actually need slides. If you do need slides, how many will you need? A complex subject might actually require fewer slides, but more time to explain the material on each slide.

You might reflect on methods of communicating your material. Is there another way to get your message across? For example, instead of lecturing on stress to house staff, one professor devised a Jeopardy game that touched on all the facts he would have presented in a lecture. Residents became more animated and competitive playing the game, and they appreciated the active learning format.

In contrast, lectures are often a passive learning experience where, to paraphrase Edwin E. Slosson,[2] the notes of the speaker become the notes of the listener without passing through the mind of either. In these situations, attending a lecture is a transcription process rather than a learning one. Consider whether you should distribute more detailed written notes instead of the standard method of copies of slides.

Although the concept of a 15-minute attention span may be an urban legend,[3] it may still be advantageous to try to incorporate more active learning activities into a lecture. Quizzes have been shown to reinforce learning.[4] Can you incorporate them into your presentation as a pretest, a posttest, or even a part of your presentation? Quizzes could be used with or without the use of audience response systems (ARS). Originally a high-cost presentation hardware adjunct, the ubiquitous smartphone can now function as an ARS via apps linked to the Internet. Many programs are free for use with small groups.[5]

It may seem obvious, but delivering a presentation is quite different than reading a chapter from a textbook. A text can provide a detailed overview, whereas a lecture may only highlight important points to remember. Speakers sometimes mistakenly try to cover all the material in an accompanying text, whereas the oral medium requires a much more focused and limited emphasis.

One strategy in planning your presentation that may be helpful is the use of a story board (**Fig. 1**). Filmmakers use this technique to help visualize the sequence of their movie. During the planning process, write talking points on sticky notes or index cards. These cards or notes may then be moved around to adjust the flow of your materials. The Slide Sorter function in PowerPoint can provide a digital alternative to the analog process of paper cards.

Augmentation

If the decision is made to use presentation software, the primary consideration should be how to use the application to enhance the message to be delivered rather than distract from it. Slides should never be scripts from which the presentation is read. They should help guide the presentation and reinforce the points to be made.

The most common mistake in preparing a slide is to include too much information or too many bullet points. The audience can read faster than the speaker can enunciate, resulting in a disconnect between the oral presentation and the material being viewed. Conversely, because slides typically are on screen for only a few moments, there may be insufficient time for the audience to comprehend a complicated slide.

For example, a graph from a textbook is meant to be viewed along with the accompanying text. The reader may move back and forth from text to diagram to understand

Story Board

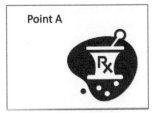
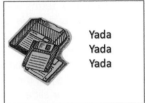
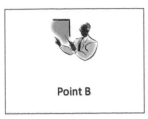

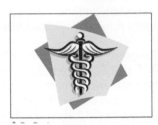
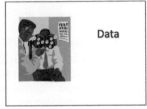
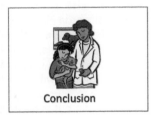

Fig. 1. Story boards allow you to plan and edit the sequence of your presentation. (*Courtesy of* Carlyle Chan, M.D. Milwaukee, Wisconsin.)

the diagram or graph's various facets. Using a complicated graph or diagram like the one in a textbook for a presentation does not permit the audience to digest it in a similar manner. It is best to simplify or highlight the portion of the image needed to emphasize the point being made.

A second mistake is overusing animations. Presentation software can offer various ways to display your bullet points. Having information fly onto the screen from different directions or otherwise dramatically appear does nothing to enhance the lecture material and becomes another distraction.

When bullet points are necessary, one useful animation technique is to apply "appear" to your bullets. Using this feature allows each point to appear in sequence as you explain each point, thus preventing the audience from their natural inclination to read ahead and not hear what you are saying. There is even an exit feature that dims the previous point, again focusing on your immediate discussion. Focus remains an integral part of the learning experience.

Multiple types of presentation software are available. PowerPoint by Microsoft is the most common. Keynote is an Apple presentation app, and there are dozens of others.[6] Prezi[7] is an animated nonlinear application that has gained popularity. These general guidelines apply to any such apps.

Death by PowerPoint is a generic phrase that has been used to describe the boredom associated with many software-assisted presentations. A Google search on the term finds 123,000,000 results. The 2003 *Columbia* shuttle craft disaster revealed that actual death, and not just being bored to death, may have resulted from a poorly constructed slide presentation.

Edward Tufte is Professor Emeritus of political science, statistics, and computer science at Yale University. He is known for his contributions in information design and data visualization. After the 2003 *Columbia* space shuttle disaster, Professor Tufte was a member of the *Columbia* Accident Investigation Board.[8] After a piece of foam insulation from the thruster rockets struck the underside of the shuttle upon takeoff, engineers had to determine whether it was safe for the shuttle to reenter the earth's atmosphere.

Engineers produced 3 reports and 28 slides. Tufte found in one slide in particular: among other things, the title was misleading, terms were vague, and contradictory information was buried in lower levels of the slide. The result was NASA officials unfortunately decided it was safe for the *Columbia* to return. The Investigation Board concluded "it was easy to understand how a senior manager might read this PowerPoint slide and not realize that it addresses a life-threatening situation." Tufte thought a written document would have better conveyed the engineers' concerns.

An Internet search reveals multiple rules for slide construction.[9,10] There are 1-5-5, 1-6-6, 1-7-7, and even 1-8-8 rules. The common feature to all is one idea per slide. Each rule varies as to the maximum of lines (5, 6, 7, or 8) per slide, and the maximum number of words (5, 6, 7, or 8) per line. However, any of these rules create slides that are text heavy (**Box 1**, **Figs. 2** and **3**).

Other approaches, such as the Takahashi method,[11,12] suggest using only one or 2 words per slide in a very large font. There is also the Godin[12] method that emphasizes the use of visuals with or without text to highlight your points and evoke an emotional connection to your point. The Lessig method[12] combines the approaches of Takahashi and Godin but expects slides to be displayed for no longer than 15 seconds. For businesses, Guy Kawasaki suggests a 10/20/30 rule for PowerPoint.[13] He recommends limiting your presentation to 10 slides, limiting to no longer than 20 minutes, and using only 30-point fonts or larger (**Box 2**, **Figs. 4–8**).

All of these techniques have one common message: Simplify your message and slides, or as the aphorism says, "Less is More."

It has been said that a picture is worth a thousand words. When inserting a photograph or image, software usually places the image within a smaller box in the middle of the slide with a title line at the top. Edward Tufte feels that this surrounding margin is a waste of space and does not convey information. Also, the image and script may not be so visible from the back of the room. It is best to expand the image to fill the entire slide area and embed any script. Be sure the image has sufficient resolution to enlarge.

Box 1
Maximum number of lines and words per slide

- Debate regarding maximum number
- Some advocate 5 lines maximum
- Limit to 5 words per line
- Other guides: 6, 7, and even 8 maximum
- Agreement on one topic per slide
- Avoid using long complete sentences
- This slide uses 8 words maximum per slide
- This is still a pretty wordy slide

Courtesy of Carlyle Chan, M.D. Milwaukee, Wisconsin.

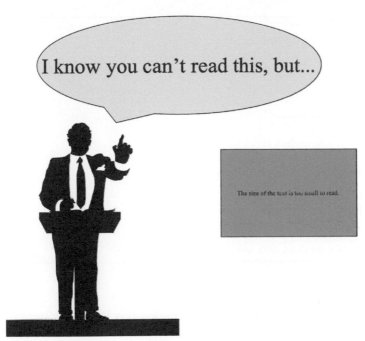

Fig. 2. Importance of font size. (*Courtesy of* Carlyle Chan, M.D, Milwaukee, Wisconsin (patterned after slide in Upjohn Pharmaceuticals Speaker Presentation Kit).)

Just as with the font size of text, the size of the photograph does matter (**Figs. 9** and **10**).

Free images may be used, particularly if there is a Creative Commons copyright, for example, search for Flickr Creative Commons. This form of copyright permits redistribution with and sometimes without proper acknowledgment. Photographs and other information under Creative Commons provide a no-cost resource to use in presentations as well as a means to distribute your presentation. There are also multiple sources of free stock photographs (**Box 3**).

Videos may be another means of conveying pertinent information. Oftentimes presenters will link to an online site to display the clip. If possible, it is best to have an actual copy of the video to embed into the presentation software. Internet access

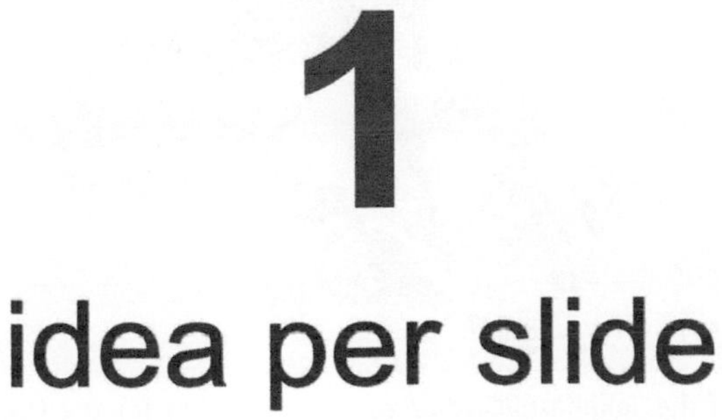

1
idea per slide

Fig. 3. Using one idea, color, and font size. (*Courtesy of* Carlyle Chan, M.D. Milwaukee, Wisconsin.)

> **Box 2**
> **Free stock photograph sites**
> - Morguefile.com
> - LifeofPix.com
> - Pixabay.com
> - Images.superfamous.com
> - StockSnap.io
> - Freestocks.org
> - Unsplash.com
> - Pexels.com
> - Negativesoace.co
> - Burst.shopifv.com
>
> *Courtesy of* Carlyle Chan, M.D. Milwaukee, Wisconsin.

and stability can be variable depending on the location of your talk and can affect the display of your video clip.

Attention to colors is important because colors can either highlight a point or, conversely, diminish the clarity of a slide. Certain color combinations can wash out the visibility of the word, whereas other combinations may clash. Also, the image on your computer screen is back lit and will likely be more intense and brighter than when it projected onto a screen in a well-lit room or auditorium. Testing color combinations in advance is important. Many speakers avoid the various available templates

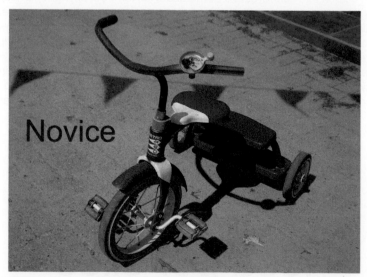

Fig. 4. Variations of the Takahashi/Godin/Lessig approaches for the Dreyfus model: novice. (*From* "Time on three wheels" by Brian Fitzgerald (https://www.flickr.com/photos/brian-fitzgerald/486954077/) is licensed under Creative Commons copyright BY 4.0.)

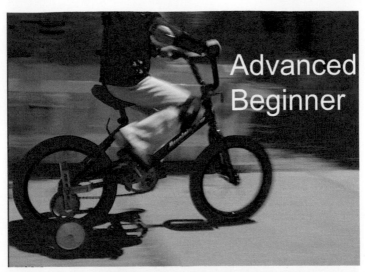

Fig. 5. Variations of the Takahashi/Godin/Lessig approaches for the Dreyfus model: advanced beginner. (*From* "zoom again" by Richo.Fan (https://www.flickr.com/photos/richo-fan/4271940123/) is licensed under Creative Commons copyright BY 4.0.)

altogether and simply use black letters on white background for text, or the reverse, white letters on black background (**Fig. 11**).

Presentation software also offers multiple options on how to create and present graphs. Graphs may take the form of lines, bars, 3-dimensional (3D) lines and bars, 3D pyramids, circles, and more. Similar to the concerns about distracting animations,

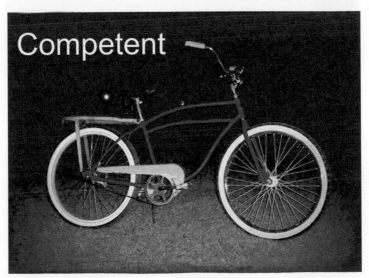

Fig. 6. Variations of the Takahashi/Godin/Lessig approaches for the Dreyfus model: competent. (*From* "Rollfast Rat Bike "Rat-n-Roll" by Arturo Sotillo (https://www.flickr.com/photos/whappen/3186403264/) is licensed under Creative Commons copyright BY 4.0.)

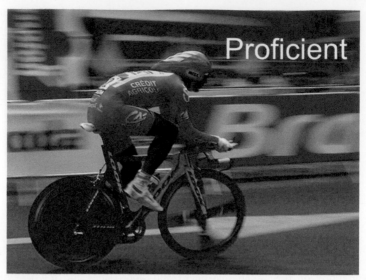

Fig. 7. Variations of the Takahashi/Godin/Lessig approaches for the Dreyfus model: proficient. (*From "Tour de France – 08"* by Celso Flors (https://www.flickr.com/photos/celso/2650518085/) is licensed under Creative Commons copyright BY 4.0.)

caution is needed so as not to violate signal-to-noise ratios. That is, fancy means of creating graphs should not obscure the intended message.

Printed copies of slides are often requested by program organizers and attendees. However, printed slides, if following the above recommendations, may be difficult to decipher in retrospect. A written summary may be a more useful handout.

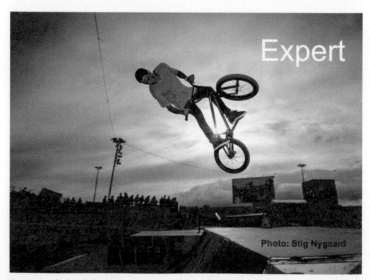

Fig. 8. Variations of the Takahashi/Godin/Lessig approaches for the Dreyfus model: expert. (*From* "BMX rider at Roskilde Festival Street City" by Stig Nygaard (https://www.flickr.com/photos/stignygaard/7500657236/) is licensed under Creative Commons copyright BY 4.0.)

CME: A Bridge to Quality

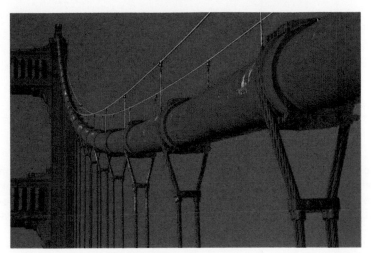

Fig. 9. Typical inserted photograph. (*Courtesy of* Carlyle Chan, M.D. Milwaukee, Wisconsin.)

Delivery

Educational researchers originally scripted a lecture to be given by an actor whom they called Dr Fox.[14] The title was "Mathematical Game Theory as Applied to Physician Education." The presentation was witty, engaging, and humorous, but utterly devoid of any factual information. Nevertheless, the speaker received high marks for his presentation. One person even claimed awareness of the speaker's nonexistent publications.

Researchers conducted a second study when they recognized that their conclusion, that style was everything, might be premature. They constructed 2 new sets of

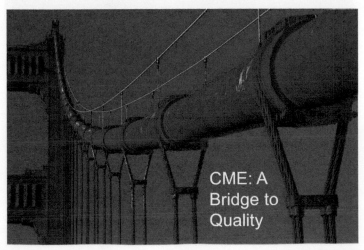

CME: A
Bridge to
Quality

Fig. 10. Expanding photograph to fill dead space and imbedding text. (*Courtesy of* Carlyle Chan, M.D. Milwaukee, Wisconsin.)

Box 3
Dreyfus Model: developmental stages of learning

- Novice
- Advanced beginner
- Competent
- Proficient
- Expert

Courtesy of Carlyle Chan, M.D. Milwaukee, Wisconsin.

---

speeches on "The Biochemistry of Learning."[15–17] One set was labeled "high-seduction" with the speaker coached to be warm and engaging, and a second set of "low-seduction" lectures, where the speaker was to deliver the material in a boring and monotone style. Each set had 3 different versions, each with 26 facts, 14 facts, and 4 facts.

A quiz was administered after each presentation based on the 26 facts. In each group, students who received a higher number of facts generally did better than students who received fewer facts. However, the group who attended the high-seduction lecture with the fewest facts did about as well as the students who attend the high-fact, low-seduction lecture. Researchers conclude that "high-seduction" presentations, as they defined it, influenced test performance even more than student ratings of speakers. Subsequent analysis also found that student incentives to learning also played a factor.[17]

Paying attention not only to what you say, but also how you say it, can contribute to a successful presentation. Some delivery styles to consider include the following.

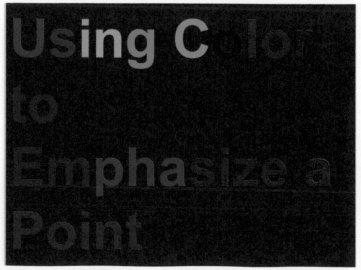

Fig. 11. Benefits and liabilities of using color. (*Courtesy of* Carlyle Chan, M.D. Milwaukee, Wisconsin.)

Passion
Part of any human interaction includes nonverbal communication. Intentionally or un-intentionally, enthusiasm or passion for your topic can be conveyed to your audience as much as disinterest in the subject matter. Monitor your level of energy as you give your talk.[18,19]

Stage presence
This is often a term reserved for performers, but it can be helpful to view a presentation as a performance. Many of the elements are the same. Rather than keeping the lectern as a barrier between you and the listeners, if equipped with a lavalier microphone, moving closer and among your audience can help establish a connection with them, assuming you have enough familiarity with your material that you need not glance at any presentation notes.[20]

Humor
Not everyone is a comedian, and even the best comedians have jokes that bomb. Humor is a way to break the ice, and if a humorous anecdote is not available, some speakers use cartoons to introduce a topic. Just be aware of copyright limitations and restrictions for fair use.

Narrative
It is important to tell a story.[21] The human brain is hardwired to remember a story better than a list of bullet points. Oral histories have predated written language. In fact, memory experts rely on stories and visual images to help them recall lists of unrelated items.[22] Working a narrative into your presentation can go a long way to assisting your learners in recalling the information presented.

Rate
Speaking too slowly or too quickly has its limitations and can influence audience disengagement. Normal conversation averages about 120 to 150 words per minute. Presentations should be similar. Listening to a recording of yourself lecturing can provide valuable feedback in determining the speed of your talk.[18] The exception is medical students, who, to save time, have learned to listen to recorded lectures at double speed.

Modulation
As noted in the Dr Fox reference, a monotone delivery can be boring. The ability to vary the modulation, inflection, and cadence of an oral presentation can assist in a more effective delivery. Examples, both good and bad, can be seen on television. TV news reporters have learned in broadcast journalism classes to modulate their voices. Television evangelists vary the intensity of their voices to hold the attention of their audiences. In contrast, some sports celebrities who endorse a product can be seen speaking in an awkward cadence.[23]

Eye contact
Looking members of the audience in the eye is a method of engaging them.[24] Rather than averting gaze or darting one's eyes from side to side, consider focusing on one audience member to deliver a single point before moving onto the next subject and listener.

Vocalized pauses
Another distraction is vocalized pauses or utterances. Saying "uhh" or "like" repeatedly can bother some in the audience. Recording a practice presentation may alert the speaker to his or her frequency of such utterances and help pay attention to suppressing them.[18,23,25]

Projection
In a large auditorium, a sound check before speaking can be beneficial, as you may need to adjust your own volume according to the sensitivity of the microphone and speaker system. In medium-sized rooms without amplification, be aware of how loudly you project. Remember to enunciate clearly.[18]

Verbal transitions
Journal articles have identified sections, such as Introduction, Methods, Results, and Conclusions. Because such sections are not readily recognized aurally, presentations benefit from auditory markers or transitions. There is an old speaking adage: "Tell them what you're going to tell them. Tell them. Tell them what you told them." Giving an audience an introduction before the main address and a summary afterward provides guidance for the listener. It is also best that if you say, "In conclusion…", to really mean it. Speakers have been known to drone on too long. These techniques are, again, to help the listener to focus on your message.

Comprehensiveness
There is a temptation is to try to cover too much in a lecture. Comprehensive detail can add to information overload. The saying, "Leave them wanting more," may not be a bad idea. Focus on the important takeaway points. Editing your talk is not unlike editing any other creative product.

Scientific meeting presentations often encounter strict time limits that may proscribe showing all the data you wish to present in the time available. One tip is to reserve some data slides after your formal presentation slides. Then, if during the question-and-answer segment a pertinent question arises, you can say, "I'm glad you asked that," and then take the opportunity to present that extra piece of information.

Practice/rehearsal
"How do you get to Carnegie Hall?" is a proverbial question. As with any performance, practice and rehearsals fine tune the actual delivery and provide an opportunity to modify content.[18] Rehearsing with a friendly audience can help with feedback and anticipate questions. With smartphones, it has also become easier to record yourself to observe and critique your own talk.

SUMMARY

The 3 elements described in this article provide a template to creating a successful presentation. Planning ahead for a talk encompasses a series of decisions deserving consideration before constructing the actual presentation. Simplified slides will support rather than distract from your message and help keep your audience connected to what you are saying. Paying attention to your delivery style will help your audience learn and retain the information you are trying to convey.

CLINICS CARE POINTS

- One main idea per slide.
- Minimize the amount of text in your slides.
- Use large fonts.
- A picture is worth a thousand words.
- Ensure that your slides enhance and not distract from your message.

- Remember to enunciate, modulate, and project if no microphone.
- Tell a story, do not read a slide or list.
- Practice, practice, practice.

DISCLOSURE

The author has nothing to disclose.

REFERENCES

1. Wisconsin Center for Educational Research. Doing collaborative learning. Available at: http://archive.wceruw.org/cl1/cl/doingcl/advlec.htm. Accessed May 24, 2020.
2. Slosson EE. Great American Universities. New York: Macmillan Company; 1910. p. 520 (Google Books full view).
3. Bradbury NA. Attention span during lectures: 8 seconds, 10 minutes or more? Adv Physiol Educ 2016;40:509–13.
4. Cook BR, Babon A. Active learning through online quizzes: better learning and less (busy) work. J Geogr Higher Educ 2017;42:1.
5. Audience Response Software. Available at: https://www.capterra.com/audience-response-software/. Accessed May 24, 2020.
6. The Best Presentation Software. Available at: https://zapier.com/blog/best-powerpoint-alternatives/. Accessed May 9, 2020.
7. Prezi. Available at: https://prezi.com. Accessed May 18, 2020.
8. Tufte E. PowerPoint does rocket science – and better techniques for technical reports. Available at: https://www.edwardtufte.com/bboard/q-and-a-fetch-msg?msg_id=0001yB. Accessed May 12, 2020.
9. What is the 5 by 5 rule in PowerPoint?. Available at: https://www.quora.com/What-is-the-5-by-5-rule-in-PowerPoint. Accessed August 25, 2020.
10. Reynolds G. Presentation zen: simple ideas on presentation design and delivery. 3rd Edition. Berkely CA: New Riders Publisher; 2020. p. 150.
11. The Takahashi method. Available at: https://www.ethos3.com/design-tips/the-takahashi-method/. Accessed May 10, 2020.
12. Schelle T. 3 presentation styles to keep your audience entertained. Available at: https://24slides.com/presentbetter/3-presentation-styles-to-keep-your-audience-entertained/. Accessed May 11, 2020.
13. Kawasaki G. The 10/20/30 rule of PowerPoint. Available at: https://guykawasaki.com/the_102030_rule/. Accessed April 10, 2020.
14. Ware J, Williams RG. The Dr. Fox effect: a study of lecturer effectiveness and ratings of instruction. J Med Educ 1975;50(2):149–56.
15. Williams RG, Ware JR. An extended visit with Dr. Fox: validity of student satisfaction with instruction ratings after repeated exposures to a lecturer. Am Educ Res J 1977;12(4):449–57.
16. Williams RG, Ware JE. Validity of student ratings of instruction under different incentive conditions: a further study of the Dr. Fox effect. J Educ Psychol 1976;68(1):48–56.
17. Marsh HW, Ware JE. Effects of expressiveness, content coverage and incentive on multidimensional student rating scales: new interpretations of the Dr. Fox effect. J Educ Psychol 1982;74(1):126–34.

18. Toastmasters International. Your speaking voice. Available at: https://www.toastmasters.org/~/media/B7D5C3F93FC3439589BCBF5DBF521132.ashx. Accessed May 16, 2020.

19. ForbesSpeakers. 5 ways of speaking passionately and with a purpose. Available at: https://forbesspeakers.com/5-ways-of-speaking-passionately-and-with-a-purpose/. Accessed May 16, 2020.

20. 9 Simple and effective public speaking tips for scientists. Scientifica NeuroWire. Available at: https://www.scientifica.uk.com/neurowire/9-simple-and-effective-public-speaking-tips-for-scientists. Access May 26, 2020.

21. Brannon A, Lomheim J. National Council of Teachers of English. The power of storytelling: using narrative to develop speaking and listening skills. Available at: https://ncte.org/blog/2020/02/the-power-of-storytelling/. Accessed May 26, 2020.

22. Foer J. Moonwalking with Einstein: the art and science of remembering everything. New York: The Penguin Press; 2011.

23. Verbal fillers in public speaking. Clemson University. Available at: https://www.clemson.edu/cbshs/departments/communication/centers/Verbal%20Fillers.pdf. Accessed May 16, 2020.

24. 10 reasons eye contact is everything in public speaking. Available at: https://www.inc.com/sims-wyeth/10-reasons-why-eye-contact-can-change-peoples-perception-of-you.html. Accessed May 16, 2020.

25. Yale Poorvu Center for teaching and learning. Available at: https://poorvucenter.yale.edu/teaching/ideas-teaching/public-speaking-teachers-ii-mechanics-speaking. Accessed May 16, 2020.

Adapting Teaching to the Clinical Setting

Jeffrey I. Hunt, MD[a],*, Elizabeth H. Brannan, MD[a], Vicenta B. Hudziak, MD[b]

KEYWORDS

- Experiential learning • Apprenticeship • Supervision • Clinical

KEY POINTS

- The apprenticeship model remains important for postgraduate medical education. Experiential learning theory is useful for understanding the apprenticeship model in the clinical setting.
- Six important tools of experiential learning are scaffolding, modeling, coaching/supervision, articulation, reflection, and exploration.
- Cultivating acceptance and nurturing change is critical for long-term success in learning in the clinical setting. It is important for supervisors to cultivate nonjudgmental acceptance of themselves for continued professional growth as supervisors.
- Supervisors in clinical settings need adequate protected time to optimally teach in the apprenticeship model

CONSIDERATIONS

The traditional apprenticeship model of medical education that follows a preclinical period of study has been in place for well over a century.[1] The apprenticeship model provides learners with an opportunity to experience authentic clinical challenges in a real-life context, and learning occurs in a process whereby "knowledge is created through the transformation of experience."[2] The apprenticeship model of learning requires supported active participation by the apprentice and for them to feel "legitimate" in their role within the team.[3,4] It is clear that in all levels of undergraduate and postgraduate training the apprenticeship model remains important and that, as suggested by Tosteson, "we must acknowledge that the most important, indeed, the only thing we have to offer our students is ourselves. Everything else they can read in a book."[5] This experiential learning process must occur within a safe setting and needs to be managed efficiently by trained supervisors. For the apprenticeship model to be successful, the team must be educated in the role of the apprentice and the apprentice made to feel a vital part of the team. This requires investment of

[a] Department of Psychiatry and Human Behavior, Alpert Medical School of Brown University, Bradley Hospital, 1011 Veterans Memorial Parkway, East Providence, RI 02915, USA; [b] Alpert Medical School of Brown University, Rhode Island Hospital POB, Suite 122, 593 Eddy Street, Providence, RI 02915, USA
* Corresponding author.
E-mail address: Jeffrey_hunt@brown.edu

Psychiatr Clin N Am 44 (2021) 197–205
https://doi.org/10.1016/j.psc.2020.12.003
0193-953X/21/© 2021 Elsevier Inc. All rights reserved.

time and resources in educating the teams involved and for mentors to be allowed protected time to dedicate to their apprentices.[6]

Clinical teaching allows for both working and learning to occur; one author described "teaching and learning being rooted in the doing of work, not just talking about it."[7] Not surprisingly, the apprenticeship model is used universally and has been ranked by residents as a highly favored method of learning, that depends on the availability of skilled and enthusiastic teachers and the appropriate quantity and mix of patients.[8] This article first discusses the apprenticeship model of learning and teaching through the experiential learning theory in the context of adapting learning to the clinical setting. We then describe the importance of the cultivation of acceptance of the learner while nurturing change in the clinical teaching environment. We describe resident reflections on learning within the clinical environments seen in pediatrics and general psychiatry as a way of highlighting these concepts. Finally, we describe the financial challenges inherent with this model and some strategies to overcome them.

UNDERSTANDING LEARNING IN THE CLINICAL SETTING: EXPERIENTIAL LEARNING THEORY

The cognitive apprenticeship framework based on experiential learning theory is useful for understanding learning in the clinical setting.[9] Feinstein and colleagues[10] have described 6 tools of experiential learning as components of this framework in the context of training in psychotherapy for residents. These tools are scaffolding, modeling, coaching/supervision, articulation, reflection, and exploration. These tools provide useful guidance for supervisors to effectively teach in the context of clinical settings (**Box 1**.).

CULTIVATING ACCEPTANCE WHILE NURTURING CHANGE IN CLINICAL TEACHING

The process of becoming a competent physician is an inherently change-driven one. Knowledge, skills, and broader competencies are iteratively obtained, practiced, and refined throughout training and one's professional career via life-long learning. At the same time, in the realm of psychotherapy, dialectical behavioral therapy and acceptance and commitment therapy, among others, teach us that the nonjudgmental acceptance of where a patient is at any given moment in the process of learning is necessary, although not alone sufficient, for further change to occur.[11,12] Although trainees are not patients and supervisors are not their therapists, a similar process of acceptance and change is applicable to any relationship and environment organized around growth and learning.

For supervisors to facilitate learning and growth in trainees, supervisors must first and continuously observe, describe, and nonjudgmentally accept where our trainees are in emotional, cognitive, and behavioral terms using some of the same experiential learning tools listed elsewhere in this article. Inherent in this process is the concept of validation. In learning how to practice dialectical behavioral therapy, therapists learn the concept of "validating the valid."[11] This process refers to learning how to acknowledge one's own or another person's feelings and thoughts and genuinely and nonjudgmentally accept them as real, legitimate, and "making sense" in the context of that person's lived experience. The therapist does not have to *agree* with them or experience them the same way to acknowledge and accept that they are true. Similarly, patients themselves learn to "self-validate" or reflect throughout the process of engaging in dialectical behavioral therapy. This applies to the training process in medical school, residency, fellowship, and beyond. Patients, and learners at any level,

> **Box 1**
> **Tools of experiential learning**
>
> - *Scaffolding* refers to teaching trainees at their individual developmental level and continuously building on the trainee's prior achievements. Support, knowledge, suggestions, and specific help are provided only when needed to address the trainee's current needs.
>
> - *Modeling* occurs when supervisors (experts) demonstrate aspects of assessment and psychotherapy techniques to residents (observers) and explain their reasoning and thought processes underlying their clinical decisions. Modeling enables the trainee not only to watch the expert, but also to subsequently demonstrate that the trainee has assimilated the techniques used by the expert in conducting the same (or similar) tasks.
>
> - *Coaching* occurs when trainees are watched performing clinical work or soon after (perhaps using in-the-room sessions, through video with blue tooth technology, or immediately after the observed session). The supervisors offer in-the-moment alternative therapeutic statements or interventions. Coaching can be combined with modeling and is tailored to the trainee's developmental trajectory. Coaching in the traditional format of weekly psychotherapy supervision occurring after the fact is enhanced by the review of video or audio and to some extent by the review of carefully documented process notes.
>
> - *Articulation* (also called Socratic questioning) describes the process by which supervisors ask trainees nonthreatening but thought-provoking questions. Supervisors can use Socratic questioning to help trainees explicitly explain their clinical reasoning as well as the emotions elicited during the encounter, including describing the transference, countertransference, or resistances in the meeting with patient. Articulation helps trainees to deepen their knowledge and improves their reflection skills. Supervisors can also use articulation to assess trainee's depth of understanding.
>
> - *Reflection* encourages trainees to individually examine their psychotherapy and clinical experiences to assess their own learning needs.
>
> - *Exploration* is supported when supervisors stimulate trainees to read and think independently about various aspects of their clinical work.
>
> *Data from* Feinstein, R.E., R. Huhn, and J. Yager, Apprenticeship Model of Psychotherapy Training and Supervision: Utilizing Six Tools of Experiential Learning. Acad Psychiatry, 2015. 39(5): p. 585-9.

are "doing the best they can" at any given moment *and* we and they want them to learn "to do better." We will struggle to effectively help them do better if we do not fully acknowledge and accept where they are now. It is through holding the frames of acceptance and change at the same time and facile movement back and forth between validating the valid and encouraging and scaffolding change that learning occurs. If we only validate and accept and do not identify what needs changing, learners do not grow or advance. In the extremes, they either develop a false sense of competence and do not know what they do not know, or they feel insecure and questioning of their legitimacy and competence as physicians.

In a seminar about giving and receiving feedback as a learner, a trainee shared with 1 author that, "I don't want to be told I'm doing great when I know I'm not." Telling a trainee that they are doing well at something they do not believe that they are doing well, even if the supervisor assesses that the trainee is meeting milestones, is invalidating and can inhibit rather than foster growth. Exploring the trainee's thoughts about where they are in their learning and the emotions brought up in that and validating them is as important as teaching new knowledge or skills and bolstering confidence. A dialectical approach a supervisor could take with this trainee would be to first ask how the trainee thinks they are doing and how they are feeling about the rotation or encounter, validating their experience of worrying or doubting themselves in this example (or feeling confident and competent in other cases), then exploring together via problem solving the areas for growth and change. Validation for the trainee who is doubtful and anxious could sound something like this: "It makes a lot of sense that you would doubt your abilities when you are being asked to learn and do so many new things in such short order while constantly being evaluated." A supervisor would not even have to go that far if they did not have an idea of why a trainee might feel that way, and instead the supervisor could say, "You're really doubting yourself and your abilities, I can see that. That is a hard way to feel." If the supervisor stopped there, the trainee may stay paralyzed with insecurity. Conversely, if the supervisor says, "You're doing great, you should be more confident," the trainee has just been invalidated, which also does not foster growth, but may contribute to apparent competence rather than true competence. Instead, to balance acceptance and change, the supervisor might say, "Even if I think your knowledge and skill level are where they should be for your level of training, I can tell that is not your experience, and that is important for us to explore. Help me understand more how you are thinking and feeling about this." From there, a dialogue can unfold that may help to elucidate potential distorted thoughts, underlying emotional experiences, or perceived skills deficits that the supervisor can help the trainee address in a process of problem solving.

An important mediating factor to consider will be the degree to which the trainee actually does need to change, for example, the trainee who is not meeting the milestones for their level of training, the trainee who is demonstrating unprofessional behavior, the trainee who is underfunctioning or overfunctioning in response to stress. Thus, there may be heavier emphasis at various points on change and problem solving, and still, before and along, with any change agenda must be acceptance and validation of what is valid.

Another important mediating factor is the supervisor's own experience with self-validating and receiving validation from others. We cannot overstate the importance of supervisors cultivating nonjudgmental acceptance of themselves while continuing to grow, reflect on, and explore their work as supervisors. The relative ability of the supervisor to self-validate and their experience with being validated can contribute to or detract from their willingness and ability to accept their trainees' experiences before and during the process of change.

A necessary part of being able to validate one's own or someone else's experience is to understand it. This point is particularly relevant for the role emotional experiences play in the learning environment. The degree to which a supervisor can effectively validate their own and their trainees' experiences will depend on the degree to which they know themselves and their trainees, respectively. This leads to the role for supervisors making time and space to intentionally engage in self-reflection and exploration as well as learning about their trainee's lived experience before and during the process of teaching them. This process can create discomfort for a host of reasons. Some may argue that this process is akin to therapy and should be the role of a trainee's therapist rather than their supervisor. Although there is undoubtedly a role for a trainee's (or supervisor's) own therapy when patterns of maladaptive thinking, feeling, or behaving are the issue, there exists a crucial place in supervision for eliciting, accepting, and effectively using the trainee's lived experience, emotions, and cognitions through reflection and exploration as they come up in relation to patient cases to help guide treatment and learning. The same point applies in the supervision process for the supervisor. Supervisors have their own lived experience, emotions, and cognitions that must be understood and considered in the process of providing supervision. Strategic self-disclosure by a supervisor to a trainee about the supervisor's own process of professional growth and learning can be powerful catalysts for change in trainees. This process requires starting from a place of acceptance and validation, and it can be uncomfortable. The authors have experiences with trainees who earnestly want their patients to be vulnerable and tolerate distress in the service of growth but who themselves struggle to do the same, which in turn can hinder the trainees' authentic and effective presence in their physician–patient relationships. Insofar as supervisors can share their own experiences of feeling and tolerating discomfort, in the form of painful emotional experiences or distressing thoughts or behavioral mistakes in relation to their work as physicians, trainees can at once feel seen and understood and learn this process experientially as outlined in the cognitive apprenticeship framework presented elsewhere in this article. Receiving nonjudgmental acceptance and validation from a supervisor can also provide powerful modeling for how to give these gifts to their patients.

A related process can occur in the context of cultural humility in supervision. The authors recently engaged in a seminar together with their senior trainees in which supervisors and trainees completed the Cultural Self-Assessment from Pamela Hays' text *Addressing Cultural Complexities in Practice* (2016).[13] Supervisors and trainees alike described to one another in depth their lived experience and influences across the 9 domains of the ADDRESSING Framework (Age and generational influences, Developmental or other Disability, Religion and spiritual orientation, Ethnic and racial identity, Socioeconomic status, Sexual orientation, Indigenous heritage, National origin, and Gender). This practice set a solid foundation for supervisors and trainees together to examine influences from their lived experience on their emotional and cognitive reactions to their patients, and this process had direct effects on supervision as well. Multiple trainees shared personal or familial experiences with mental illnesses, racism, and structural inequities that they had never discussed with their supervisors but that inevitably were bringing up complex emotions in their work with patients, and this work allowed subsequent supervisors to be mindful of these reactions and help trainees navigate them. Additionally, we believe as supervisors that our own willingness to be vulnerable by self-disclosing the details of our lived experience with our trainees helped to model and scaffold for our trainees how to do the same.

SUCCESSES AND CHALLENGES OF APPRENTICESHIP: A TRAINEE PERSPECTIVE

While in residency, it is challenging to step back and reflect on the process of becoming a physician. Amid the unforgiving pace and relative chaos of the first 2 years, mentors become a critical anchor for trainees. The apprenticeship model is truly gratifying in the supervisor–trainee relationship in which the supervisor is themselves genuinely passionate, confident, self-aware, and vulnerable, which trainees immediately detect and gravitate toward. The positive impact of cultivating acceptance and nurturing change is far reaching and begins during the intern year. For appropriate growth in residency and patient safety, it is crucial that residents gain comfort with stating what they do not know, acknowledging vulnerability, and demonstrate a willingness to admit mistakes. However, this is a major hurdle for interns to overcome as they transition from the role of fourth-year medical student who in most settings was not accustomed to any of these practices. In my experience, it was the supervisors who themselves stated "I don't know, let's find out together," acknowledged their own emotional response to a tense or tragic patient encounter, and made it clear when they made a mistake, who empowered me to drop the fourth-year medical student practice of worrying alone about knowing everything, and to start worrying with others about not knowing very much. It was nothing short of liberating.

Although gratified to start practicing medicine, trainees eventually transition to leading a team, and are then faced with the crippling fear of doing something wrong. At this stage, growth emerges necessarily only after a certain amount of experience, but also only in the setting of working with supervisors who have understood how to nurture change. These are the supervisors who are able to teach how to be "comfortable with discomfort." This goal is achieved again through the process of scaffolding, modeling, coaching, and articulation. In pediatrics, repetitive, Socratic questioning about ventilator management on rounds in the neonatal intensive care unit slowly cultivates a familiarity with a once completely alien process. Supervisors make clear what is dangerous, what is safe, and where there is room for "the art of medicine." Those supervisors who elicit feedback from their own peers about their clinical decisions and frequently debrief patient encounters, model for trainees the richness and value inherent in truly practicing medicine as a team. In psychiatry, we are encouraged to assess our emotional response to every patient, face the reality of our relative dearth of understanding of the main organ we treat and the associated pharmacology, and initially rely heavily on our supervisors to develop boundaries, style, and diagnostic skill. Seeing patients together offers an invaluable opportunity to hear in real time a supervisor's thought process, which may, for example, illuminate to a trainee why what they perceived to be callous was actually clinically indicated, thereby making us more flexible thinkers in a brief but profound moment. In all, the result for trainees is another powerful realization, that we can be uncomfortable, and still make a good decision, so that the first time we are alone and asked to change a ventilator setting for a premature infant in the neonatal intensive care unit, or are faced with the decision to prescribe a potent antipsychotic on inpatient psychiatry, we miraculously know what to do; and if we do not, know exactly who to ask.

With the advent of the current pandemic, trainees and supervisors have found themselves torn apart and separated by screens and phones and at the mercy of wireless connectivity. Conducting pediatric well-child visits over the phone, interviewing psychotic patients in a psychiatric intensive care unit over a Zoom call, and providing support for those with substance use disorders in a partial hospital program over a Zoom call and the telephone has brought with it a significantly higher burden of time and coordination for supervisors when they are in person and the trainees are not. This remote process has dramatically decreased the ability to experience the energy "in the room," and greatly heightened the challenges associated with coordination of care that would normally be accomplished by multidisciplinary rounds with many staff members present. Despite all of these obstacles, there is an inherent intensity and intimacy of interaction when participating in supervision with a supervisor face to face on a Zoom call (likely at a makeshift desk in your kitchen), and in the brief time of telehealth thus far there have been many rewarding interactions. This shift has led supervisors to teach with greater intention, and patient interactions have been enriched by many patients' relative greater comfort with technology than in-person interaction. The future of telehealth and how the apprenticeship model will thrive in that realm or not remains uncertain, and we are confident that, together, supervisors and trainees will adapt for the better and for the well-being of our patients.

THE APPRENTICE MODEL AND THE NEED FOR PROTECTED TIME

It is clear that the cognitive apprentice model is highly regarded by trainees and supervisors alike. It is also evident that there is a cost to "offering our students ourselves," as Tosteson has encouraged.[5] Skeff and colleagues[14] point out that teaching is time consuming when done well because it includes planning, instructing, and reflecting. They argued that, for teaching to be optimal, it is more than just giving advice regarding clinical care and requires the crucial step of guiding the learners to ask new questions (explore) and think critically and creatively (reflect).[14] Brenner and colleagues[15] appropriately point out that the longstanding issue of whether and how to protect time for faculty to teach in this optimal manner is very challenging. The ability for faculty to engage their students on clinical services in the manner described elsewhere in this article is clearly limited by excessive workloads, including the excessive size of patient panels and a lack of time for individual patients, diminished reimbursements, greater bureaucratic demands, and, thus, an overall decrease in what physicians actually find personally rewarding.[16,17] For academic physicians, time for education has been shown to enhance meaning in work and increases overall professional satisfaction.[18,19] Several ideas have been promoted by Brenner and colleagues[15] to address how institutions could protect the time needed for academic and clinical faculty to teach. They have advocated for academic medical center systems to develop plans to ensure that clinical teaching and supervision is protected and rewarded. They propose that there be allocation of salary support for specific teaching tasks or that the teaching faculty member's clinical productivity requirements can be decreased when supervising medical students and residents in the clinic or inpatient service.[14] Having success in protection of the faculty member's time for teaching ensures that the apprenticeship model described elsewhere in this article will thrive.

SUMMARY

Adapting teaching to the clinical setting is most successful when the teacher and trainee are able to work alongside of each other allowing the cognitive apprenticeship model to be embraced. Six tools of experiential learning as components of this framework are described in this article, including scaffolding, modeling, coaching/supervision, articulation, reflection, and exploration. These tools provide useful guidance for supervisors to effectively teach in the context of clinical settings. This experiential learning process must occur within a safe setting and needs to be efficiently managed by trained supervisors. The process of becoming a competent physician is an inherently change-driven one. Knowledge, skills, and broader competencies are iteratively obtained, practiced, and refined throughout training and one's professional career via life-long learning. For supervisors to facilitate learning and growth in trainees, supervisors must first and continuously observe, describe, and nonjudgmentally accept where our trainees are in emotional, cognitive, and behavioral terms. Inherent in this process is the concept of validation of the trainees and includes the importance of supervisors cultivating nonjudgmental acceptance of themselves while continuing to grow, reflect and explore their work as supervisors. For appropriate growth in residency and patient safety, it is crucial that residents gain comfort with stating what they do not know, acknowledging vulnerability, and demonstrate a willingness to admit mistakes. This development requires an investment of time and resources in educating the teams involved and for mentors to be allowed protected time to dedicate to their apprentices. Surveys of clinical teachers have demonstrated that the stipend was not the strongest motivator or source of satisfaction instead, but that decreasing the financial stress allowed space for the revitalizing experience of meaningful work as an educator.[20]

CLINICS CARE POINTS

- The traditional apprenticeship model of medical education has been in place for well over a century. This experiential learning process in medicine must occur within a safe setting and needs to be efficiently managed by trained supervisors.

- The apprenticeship model of learning in the clinical setting is best understood through the experiential learning theory. Important tools within experiential learning include scaffolding, modeling, coaching/supervision, articulation, reflection, and exploration.

- To facilitate learning and growth in trainees, supervisors must first and continuously observe, describe, and nonjudgmentally accept where our trainees are in emotional, cognitive, and behavioral terms and also model their own vulnerabilities.

- For appropriate growth to occur for trainees, it is crucial that they gain comfort with stating what they do not know, acknowledging vulnerability, and demonstrate a willingness to admit mistakes. Supervisors model for trainees the richness and value inherent in practicing medicine as a team

- Teaching in the clinical setting is time consuming when done well because it includes planning, instructing, and reflecting. Academic medical center systems need to develop plans to ensure that clinical teaching and supervision is protected and rewarded.

DISCLOSURE

J.I. Hunt: Honorarium from John Wiley Publishers, Grant support from NIMH. E.H. Brannan and V.B. Hudziak: none.

REFERENCES

1. Dornan T. Osler, Flexner, apprenticeship and 'the new medical education. J R Soc Med 2005;98(3):91–5.
2. Kolb. Experiential learning: experience as a source of learning and development. Englewood Cliffs (NJ): Prentice Hall; 1984.
3. Dornan T, Boshuizen H, King N, et al. Experience-based learning: a model linking the processes and outcomes of medical students' workplace learning. Med Educ 2007;41(1):84–91.
4. Morris C. Facilitating learning in the workplace. Br J Hosp Med (Lond) 2010; 71(1):48–50.
5. Tosteson DC. Learning in medicine. N Engl J Med 1979;301(13):690–4.
6. Ashley EA. Medical education - beyond tomorrow? The new doctor - Asclepiad or Logiatros? Med Educ 2000;34(6):455–9.
7. Pratt DD, Arseneau R, Collins JB. Reconsidering "good teaching" across the continuum of medical education. J Contin Educ Health Prof 2001;21(2):70–81.
8. Zisook S, Benjamin S, Balon R, et al. Alternate methods of teaching psychopharmacology. Acad Psychiatry 2005;29(2):141–54.
9. Stalmeijer RE, Dolmans DH, Snellen-Balendong HA, et al. Clinical teaching based on principles of cognitive apprenticeship: views of experienced clinical teachers. Acad Med 2013;88(6):861–5.
10. Feinstein RE, Huhn R, Yager J. Apprenticeship model of psychotherapy training and supervision: utilizing six tools of experiential learning. Acad Psychiatry 2015; 39(5):585–9.
11. MacPherson HA, Cheavens JS, Fristad MA. Dialectical behavior therapy for adolescents: theory, treatment adaptations, and empirical outcomes. Clin Child Fam Psychol Rev 2013;16(1):59–80.
12. Coyne LW, McHugh L, Martinez ER. Acceptance and commitment therapy (ACT): advances and applications with children, adolescents, and families. Child Adolesc Psychiatr Clin N Am 2011;20(2):379–99.

13. Hays PA. Addressing cultural complexities in practice : assessment, diagnosis, and therapy. 3rd edition. Washington, DC: American Psychological Association. vii; 2016. p. 355.
14. Skeff KM, Bowen JL, Irby DM. Protecting time for teaching in the ambulatory care setting. Acad Med 1997;72(8):694–7 [discussion: 693].
15. Brenner AM, Beresin EV, Coverdale JH, et al. Time to teach: addressing the pressure on faculty time for education. Acad Psychiatry 2018;42(1):5–10.
16. Shanafelt TD, Dyrbye LN, West CP. Addressing physician burnout: the way forward. JAMA 2017;317(9):901–2.
17. Krasner MS, Epstein RM, Beckman H, et al. Association of an educational program in mindful communication with burnout, empathy, and attitudes among primary care physicians. JAMA 2009;302(12):1284–93.
18. Shanafelt TD. Enhancing meaning in work: a prescription for preventing physician burnout and promoting patient-centered care. JAMA 2009;302(12):1338–40.
19. Pololi LH, Evans AT, Civian JT, et al. Faculty vitality-surviving the challenges facing academic health centers: a national survey of medical faculty. Acad Med 2015;90(7):930–6.
20. Peters AS, Schnaidt KN, Zivin K, et al. How important is money as a reward for teaching? Acad Med 2009;84(1):42–6.

Teaching Psychotherapy

Erin M. Crocker, MD[a],*, Adam M. Brenner, MD[b]

KEYWORDS

- Psychotherapy • Training • Residency • Psychiatry • Supervision

KEY POINTS

- Psychotherapy training within psychiatry residency programs has changed dramatically over the past 70 years.
- The Accreditation Council for Graduate Medical Education (ACGME) identifies supportive psychotherapy, cognitive behavioral therapy, and psychodynamic psychotherapy as the core modalities for psychotherapy training within psychiatry residency programs.
- The Psychiatry Milestones provide a framework for evaluating residents' development of psychotherapy competencies, focusing on both medical knowledge and patient care.
- A strong foundation in psychotherapy is of critical importance for preparing psychiatry residents for independent practice, regardless of their eventual practice setting.
- The American Association of Directors of Psychiatry Residency Training (AADPRT) Psychotherapy Committee has developed several resources for psychotherapy supervisors to assess residents' performance providing psychotherapy.

INTRODUCTION

Training in psychotherapy is a core element of psychiatric residency education and a vital part of our trainees' preparation for independent clinical practice. The Accreditation Council for Graduate Medical Education (ACGME) identifies supportive psychotherapy, cognitive behavioral therapy (CBT), and psychodynamic psychotherapy as the core modalities of therapy in which psychiatric residents must gain competence in order to graduate from residency and be prepared for board certification. Many studies demonstrate the efficacy of these forms of treatment and also demonstrate the importance of the fundamental abilities that are central to psychotherapy in the effective practice of pharmacotherapy. Despite this, there continues to be debate and controversy surrounding the importance of training in these vital skillsets for psychiatrists.

[a] Department of Psychiatry, University of Iowa Hospitals and Clinics, 200 Hawkins Drive, Iowa City, IA 52242, USA; [b] Department of Psychiatry, University of Texas Southwestern Medical Center, 5323 Harry Hines Boulevard, Dallas, TX 75390, USA
* Corresponding author.
E-mail address: erin-crocker@uiowa.edu

Psychiatr Clin N Am 44 (2021) 207–216
https://doi.org/10.1016/j.psc.2020.12.004
0193-953X/21/© 2020 Elsevier Inc. All rights reserved.

DEFINITIONS

Psychotherapy has been defined as a healing relationship between therapist and patient, which occurs within a structured and usually time-limited series of interactions in which the therapist uses words to provide psychological healing for the patient. This treatment occurs within a predictable healing environment that includes a clear, consistent, and predictable set of boundaries known as the therapeutic frame.[1]

The gold standard for psychotherapy training is didactic coursework along with a supervised clinical experience.[2] Psychotherapy supervision has been defined as "learning in the context of a relationship",[3] and "has long been recognized as a (if not *the*) chief means by which the traditions, practice and culture of psychotherapy are taught, transmitted, and perpetuated."[4]

HISTORY AND BACKGROUND

Psychotherapy training within psychiatry residency has changed dramatically over the past 70 years. In the middle of the twentieth century, training focused largely on psychodynamic psychotherapy and commonly included about 3000 hours of psychoanalytically oriented training.[5] By the 1990s, training in psychotherapy had been reduced within residency training programs to an average of about 200 to 600 hours total, consistent with recommendations in a 1990 Joint Taskforce Report from the Association for Academic Psychiatry (AAP) and the American Association of Directors of Psychiatric Residency Training (AADPRT).[6]

In 2001, the Accreditation Council for Graduate Medical Education (ACGME) required training residents to competence in brief, CBT, combined, psychodynamic, and supportive psychotherapies, and an expectation that trainees provide a range of individual, family, and group therapies.[7] The ACGME then revised these expectations in 2007 by prioritizing a focus on supportive, CBT, and psychodynamic as the core modalities within residency training, with an expectation that residents have "exposure" to family, group, and couples therapies.[8]

In 2013, the ACGME implemented the Milestones Project in collaboration with the American Board of Psychiatry and Neurology (ABPN); the milestones provided a framework for assessing and evaluating residents' progress in the development of various competencies, including the provision of psychotherapy. The Psychotherapy Milestones include performance expectations for residents in terms of both their medical knowledge and their patient care, as it relates to the provision of psychotherapy.[9] In 2020, the Psychiatry Milestones were updated for the reported purposes of simplicity of use, with the content of the threads reduced and with the creation of a "supplemental guide" to assist programs with evaluation of their residents using this updated version of the Psychiatry Milestones. This version retains the general categories of evaluation of medical knowledge and patient care.

CLINICAL RELEVANCE

A strong foundation in the core principles and behaviors of psychotherapy is vital within the practice behavior of psychiatrists, regardless of treatment setting. In fact, there is increasingly an understanding that all health care providers can benefit from these skillsets to some degree. It has been argued that "all clinicians could benefit from a basic understanding of psychotherapy. Medical students, therefore, should be given an opportunity to learn basic principles" of psychotherapy.[10] In addition, "simple techniques of supportive therapy can be taught to family practitioners, are appropriate for many of their patients, and can be integrated into a busy practice."[11]

The reality is that providing the best care to our patients requires a solid foundation in these abilities, because even those providers choosing to focus primarily on pharmacotherapeutic treatment interventions will be less helpful to their patients without a strong foundation in the principles and practice of psychotherapy. Various psychological factors that affect the outcome of pharmacotherapeutic intervention (including neuroticism, defensive style, locus of control, attachment style, ambivalence about medications, and readiness for change) have been summarized in detail elsewhere[12]; a provider who is not adequately prepared to respond appropriately and effectively to the specific patient within the treatment dyad, and their individualized needs, will ultimately have poorer patient outcomes.

There is evidence in the literature for the importance of these skills and abilities within general psychiatric practice. Communication and the therapeutic alliance has been shown to affect adherence to treatment in psychiatry,[13] and the alliance also affects overall patient outcomes with pharmacotherapy.[14] It has also been demonstrated that not all psychiatrists are equally effective when they prescribe medication; in fact, who we are, and how we are with the patient, has been shown to be more important in determining patient outcomes than what we ultimately prescribe.[15]

This is especially true for complex patients, where pharmacotherapy is often of little benefit unless integrated with effective psychotherapeutic interventions.[16] In fact, complex cases likely result in cost savings when both pharmacotherapy and psychotherapy are provided by the psychiatrist, compared with a split model of care, because these patients tend to be among the highest utilizers of health care services.[16,17] As we move forward as a profession we need studies that help identify which kinds of patients and circumstances specifically benefit from a psychiatrist providing both aspects of care.

CONTROVERSIES

Despite this, practice of psychotherapy by psychiatrists is threatened due to a variety of factors, including changes in reimbursement and an increase in managed care.[18,19] Survey data from 1996 through 2005 showed a significant decrease in the number of outpatient psychiatrists providing psychotherapy.[18] Importantly, data from this same survey also showed a simultaneous increase in the total number of medications prescribed at each visit within outpatient psychiatric practice.[20] We do not believe the simultaneous diminishing of psychotherapy practice by psychiatrists and the increase in polypharmacy to be a coincidence. The practice of psychotherapy fosters a nuanced understanding of each individual patient and his or her specific needs and patterns of interpersonal behaviors and coping strategies. Without this context, pharmacotherapy may be used as a very blunt and imprecise instrument with which to attempt to promote meaningful change and improvement for our patients.

A decrease in exposure to psychotherapy for residents and early career psychiatrists can indeed diminish what we are able to offer our patients, and therefore, there has been a call not only to preserve the integrity of psychotherapy training within residency programs but also to increase the focus on our residents' development of this critical and fundamental skillset.[21] As astutely noted by Gabbard and Crisp-Han, "Hippocrates is said to have asserted that 'it is more important to know the person with the illness than the illness the person has.' This ancient wisdom is no less applicable to today's patient." Therefore, it is absolutely critical for our profession to "avoid a descent into biological reductionism" and remain the "integrators *par excellence* of the biopsychosocial model of medical practice" who are able to meet the comprehensive treatment needs of our patients.[22]

NATURE OF THE PROBLEM

Survey data from training programs reiterates the need for increased focus and attention on our residents' development of these skills. A national survey of psychiatry residency programs revealed that psychodynamic psychotherapy had the greatest number of hours for didactic teaching and clinical supervision (compared with CBT and supportive therapy) but still became less than the bar set for training hours in a model curriculum developed by AADPRT and AAP. In addition, although supportive therapy was the most widely practiced form of therapy, it received the fewest teaching hours in terms of both didactic coursework and clinical supervision.[23] In a survey of residents within 15 psychiatry training programs, 28% of respondents reported concern about the adequacy of resources and time dedicated to psychotherapy training within their residency program, and about one-third of respondents felt that their program directors supported their psychotherapy training but other senior leaders in their department did not.[24] Sadly, as psychotherapy practice by psychiatrists is threatened, so too is the support and development of psychiatrists to serve as psychotherapy supervisors for our trainees,[21] and a decreased or inadequate supply of trained teachers and supervisors presents a significant barrier to adequate psychotherapy training.[21,25]

Another challenge is the absence of an international consensus on which types of psychotherapy should be prioritized within psychiatry residency training.[26] Some advocate for an increased focus on teaching manualized therapy approaches whose evidence-base is more often acknowledged in academic circles.[27,28] However, some of the studies supporting those manualized therapies commonly acknowledged to be "evidence-based" warrant careful review and interpretation, including close examination for the adequacy of the comparator therapy and for a meaningful clinical significance of results in addition to statistical significance.[29] It is also important to remember that experts and the most effective therapists use and borrow interventions from various types of therapy in a flexible manner in order to best meet the needs of each individual patient. Therefore, concerns have been expressed that adhering to manualized approaches oversimplifies the case and reduces the trainee's attunement to the patient and their ability to remain spontaneous and flexible, skills that are a vital part of the development of a fully competent therapist.[30] In addition, when discussing the evidence base for various forms of therapy, we should not forget that psychodynamic psychotherapy has been shown equally efficacious as therapies that are routinely acknowledged to be "evidence-based,"[31,32] yet this form of therapy is often not regarded as such.[32,33]

GUIDELINES

As mentioned previously, since 2007 the core modalities of psychotherapy in which our residents must achieve competence per the ACGME have been identified as supportive, CBT, and psychodynamic,[8] and these are similarly reflected in the Psychiatry Milestones.

APPROACH

Multiple approaches have been proposed for training programs to develop their residents' competency to provide the 3 core modalities of psychotherapy per ACGME. Because teaching multiple types of psychotherapy at once overwhelms learners,[34] one common approach is to start with most basic framework for therapy such as supportive psychotherapy, then move on to CBT, and then to psychodynamic psychotherapy, which is arguably the most complex and challenging framework.[35,36]

Similarly, the Y-Model of psychotherapy training has been proposed, in which common elements of psychotherapy and supportive psychotherapy are placed on the stem of the Y, and the specific competencies of CBT and psychodynamic psychotherapy are each placed on one of the branches of the Y.[37] Some approaches endeavor to teach residents to focus on the patient's needs and not initially on any particular theory or type of therapy.[35,38] Within the Psychotherapy Scholars Track at the University of Colorado, training focuses on the common elements of all therapies before discussing any specific theoretic orientation or type of therapy.[39] The psychiatry residency training program at Columbia University uses a course called "Differential Psychotherapeutics," which provides a clear rubric in which the initial steps of learning about the patient and thinking about what problems exist and what needs to change are placed well before the step of treatment-matching or beginning to consider which specific therapies could be most effective for that individual patient.[38]

OBSERVATION

Because the gold standard for psychotherapy training is composed of didactic coursework along with supervised clinical experiences,[2] a "Course and Lab" model for psychotherapy supervision has been proposed, which seeks to improve the integration between these 2 components of residents' psychotherapy training experience. This model encourages psychotherapy supervisors to keep updated on the current content of their supervisee's psychotherapy didactic coursework, such that those concepts being presented in the "course" are also examined, discussed, and evaluated by the supervisor as he or she is reviewing the resident's work in the "lab" of actual clinical experience.[40]

In general, there are noted to be 4 different overall methods of psychotherapy supervision: traditional "case discussion", co-therapy, "direct supervision with delayed feedback" (which uses video, audio, or a 1-way mirror), and live supervision using a "bug in ear" approach where the supervisor provides real-time instruction to the supervisee during a session.[41–43] The traditional approach of case discussion has the limitation of the trainees' work not being objectively observed by the supervisor; it has been noted that "therapist competence is enhanced if supervisors provide feedback on actual session material... on audio or video recordings, rather than simply discussing case material in the traditional sense".[36,44]

Unfortunately, information on which methods are actually used for supervision within training programs is both sparse and dated. A Canadian survey showed that few programs regularly used direct observation within supervision,[45] and a survey of US programs shows only 10% of supervisors using audio or video.[46]

Within supervision, residents are more open with their uncertainties if their teachers and supervisors are willing to share their struggles.[47] Areas of clinical performance that are in need of remediation can be effectively addressed using a microcounseling approach of modeling, rehearsal, and feedback.[48] This approach has been shown to help trainees improve their psychotherapy skills.[26]

ASSESSMENT AND EVALUATION

As noted earlier, residents' work in psychotherapy must be directly observed and objectively assessed if we are to ensure the development of their competence as a therapist. The sparse and dated information outlined earlier indicates that trainees in North America may not have their work as therapists directly assessed and evaluated on a regular basis. However, the use of therapy rating scales and feedback tools are a supervision best-practice.[3] Fortunately, there are many resources available that can fill this training gap. Many of these have been developed as work products of the

American Association of Directors of Psychiatric Residency Training (AADPRT) Psychotherapy Committee and are available on the AADPRT Virtual Training Office (VTO) Website at https://www.aadprt.org/training-directors/virtual-training-office.

The AADPRT Milestones Assessment for Psychotherapy, or A-MAP, provides residents and supervisors with a framework for assessment and timely feedback of common elements within the residents' psychotherapy performance, specifically assessing the use of empathy, the development of the therapeutic alliance, and the appropriate management of boundaries. The A-MAP encourages residents to select a 15-min segment of therapy video, which they believe demonstrates their best work, and the A-MAP is composed of 2 major activities. The first portion entails the selected segment of video being shown within a supervision session, whereas the supervisor uses anchor points on the A-MAP rating scale to assess performance, as it relates to empathy, alliance, and boundaries. The second portion of the A-MAP exercise includes a series of structured questions from the supervisor on the topics of empathy, alliance, and boundaries, in which the resident's responses are also rated by the supervisor. Once these 2 activities are completed, residents receive feedback on their performance in both sections. Importantly, the A-MAP can be completed during a typical 1-hour supervision session, making it an accessible tool for supervisors.

The AADPRT Supportive Therapy Rating Scales (ASTRS) provide a resource for dedicated psychotherapy supervisors, as well as general psychiatry faculty members, to observe brief supportive psychotherapy being provided by residents in all patient care settings, and can be used as an instrument to provide residents timely feedback about their performance. Faculty members who do not consider themselves to be experts in psychotherapy can realistically make use of these rating scales to evaluate the brief supportive therapy interventions being provided by residents during team rounds on inpatient psychiatric units or the consult liaison service. Dedicated psychotherapy supervisors can also make use of these rating scales within supervision when therapy recordings are available for review. There are 2 versions of the AADPRT Supportive Therapy Rating Scale: the ASTRS-A focuses on the general attitudes and approach of the resident in their supportive psychotherapy work, whereas the ASTRS-S focuses on the use of specific skills and techniques of supportive psychotherapy. In addition, there is also an AADPRT Supportive Therapy Guided Discussion exercise, in which supervisors present a series of questions focused on the resident's conceptualization of the case from a supportive psychotherapy perspective.

The AADPRT Psychodynamic Psychotherapy Rating Scales follow a similar format to the supportive therapy rating scales and offer similar advantages. These rating scales also offer 2 formats: the "Priorities" version focuses on general elements of psychodynamic psychotherapy and provides an opportunity for faculty to rate the use of these while reviewing the resident's work. The "Intervention" version focuses on the use of specific psychodynamic techniques within the session. These rating scales can serve as a resource for faculty development for supervisors and can also be of great utility in helping more junior supervisors to structure their feedback and supervision of their supervisee's work in providing psychodynamic psychotherapy.

The AADPRT Psychotherapy Committee has not developed resources for assessing performance in CBT, because the Cognitive Therapy Rating Scale (CTRS) provides a useful resource for this purpose.

DISCUSSION

Psychotherapy training within psychiatry residency has changed dramatically over the past 70 years, from an initial heavy focus on psychoanalytically oriented training to the current approach of prioritizing competence in the provision of supportive psychotherapy, CBT, and psychodynamic psychotherapy. There are a wide variety of topics of debate within the realm of psychotherapy training in psychiatry residency programs, including not only what types of therapy we should teach and how we should teach it but also regarding whether we should even be teaching these skillsets to psychiatric physicians. We believe that the fundamentals of psychotherapy are absolutely critical to the effective practice of psychiatry and that to erode this foundation from training is to diminish our ability to serve our patients in an integrative and highly effective manner. As noted earlier, as the practice of psychotherapy by psychiatrists has decreased, polypharmacy has increased. Our interpretation of these events is simple: when we do not know the patient in a meaningful way, we are more likely to use the prescription pad when a psychosocial intervention might better address the problem. For the safety and health of our patients, and for the continued integrity of our field and what we have to offer our patients, psychotherapy training must remain an extremely high priority within residency training programs for psychiatric physicians.

SUMMARY

Training in psychotherapy is a fundamental part of psychiatry residency and is vital to our trainees' preparation for independent practice. Despite financial pressures posing a threat to the practice of psychotherapy by psychiatrists, it remains of vital importance that we continue to offer our patients the comprehensive biopsychosocial care, which our training as psychiatrists uniquely prepares us to provide when we are functioning at what is truly the "top of our license" as psychiatrists. For the future of our profession and all that it has to offer patients, it is imperative that we not only preserve the integrity of psychotherapy training within psychiatry residency but that we in fact bring a renewed focus and intention to providing the highest quality of psychotherapy training possible to our resident physicians.

CLINICS CARE POINTS

- Communication and the therapeutic alliance predict outcome in pharmacotherapy.
- As psychiatrists have practiced less psychotherapy, polypharmacy has increased.
- We must provide robust training in psychotherapy to our resident physicians in order for our field to maintain all that it has to offer patients.
- Didactic coursework and a supervised clinical experience are the gold standard for psychotherapy training.
- Supportive psychotherapy, CBT, and psychodynamic psychotherapy are the core modalities of therapy per the ACGME.
- Review of objective performance data within supervision, such as therapy tapes, is vital for assessing competency and providing meaningful feedback.
- The AADPRT Psychotherapy Committee has developed numerous accessible tools for training programs and supervisors to assess their residents' work providing psychotherapy.

DISCLOSURE

Dr E.M. Crocker has nothing to disclose. Dr A.M. Brenner receives a stipend as Editor of Academic Psychiatry.

REFERENCES

1. Frank JD, Frank JB. Persuasion and healing. Baltimore (MD): Hopkins University Press; 1991.
2. Weissman MM, Verdeli H, Gameroff MJ, et al. National survey of psychotherapy training in psychiatry, psychology, and social work. Arch Gen Psychiatry 2006; 63(8):925–34.
3. Crocker EM, Sudak DM. Making the most of psychotherapy supervision: A guide for psychiatry residents. Acad Psychiatry 2017;41(1):35–9.
4. Watkins CE Jr, Scaturo DJ. Toward an integrative, learning-based model of psychotherapy supervision: Supervisory alliance, educational interventions, and supervisee learning/relearning. J Psychotherapy Integration 2013;23(1):75.
5. Giordano FL, Briones DF. Assessing residents' competence in psychotherapy. Acad Psychiatry 2003;27(3):145–7.
6. Mohl PC, Lomax J, Tasman A, et al. Psychotherapy training for the psychiatrist of the future. Am J Psychiatry 1990;147(1):7–13.
7. Miller SI, Scully JH, Winstead DK. The evolution of core competencies in psychiatry. Acad Psychiatry 2003;27(3):128–30.
8. ACGME. ACGME program requirements for graduate medical education in psychiatry. Retrieved July. 2007;1:2012. Available at: https://www.acgme.org/Portals/0/PFAssets/ProgramRequirements/400_Psychiatry_2020.pdf?ver=2020-06-19-123110-817.
9. ACGME. The psychiatry milestone project: a joint initiative of the Accreditation Council for Graduate Medical Education and the American Board of Psychiatry and Neurology 2013. Available at: https://www.acgme.org/acgmeweb/Portals/0/PDFs/Milestones/PsychiatryMilestones.pdf.
10. Truong A, Wu P, Diez-Barroso R, et al. What Is the Efficacy of Teaching Psychotherapy to Psychiatry Residents and Medical Students? Acad Psychiatry 2015; 39(5):575–9.
11. Rockland LH. A review of supportive psychotherapy, 1986-1992. Psychiatr Serv 1993;44(11):1053–60.
12. Mintz DL, Flynn DF. How (not what) to prescribe: Nonpharmacologic aspects of psychopharmacology. Psychiatr Clin 2012;35(1):143–63.
13. Thompson L, McCabe R. The effect of clinician-patient alliance and communication on treatment adherence in mental health care: a systematic review. BMC Psychiatry 2012;12(1):87.
14. Krupnick J, Sotsky S, Simmens S, et al. The role of the therapeutic alliance in psychotherapy and pharmacotherapy outcome: Findings in the NIMH Treatment of Depression Collaborative Research Program. J Consult Clin Psychol 1996; 64(3):532.
15. McKay KM, Imel ZE, Wampold BE. Psychiatrist effects in the psychopharmacological treatment of depression. J Affect Disord 2006;92(2–3):287–90.
16. Alfonso CA, Michael MC, Elvira SD, et al. Innovative educational initiatives to train psychodynamic psychiatrists in underserved areas of the world. Psychiatr Clin 2018;41(2):305–18.
17. Dewan M. Are psychiatrists cost-effective? An analysis of integrated versus split treatment. Am J Psychiatry 1999;156(2):324–6.
18. Mojtabai R, Olfson M. National trends in psychotherapy by office-based psychiatrists. Arch Gen Psychiatry 2008;65(8):962–70.
19. Olfson M, Marcus SC, Pincus HA. Trends in office-based psychiatric practice. Am J Psychiatry 1999;156(3):451–7.

20. Mojtabai R, Olfson M. National trends in psychotropic medication polypharmacy in office-based psychiatry. Arch Gen Psychiatry 2010;67(1):26–36.
21. Kay J, Myers MF. Current state of psychotherapy training: Preparing for the future. Psychodynamic psychiatry 2014;42(3):557–73.
22. Gabbard GO, Crisp-Han H. The early career psychiatrist and the psychotherapeutic identity. Acad Psychiatry 2017;41(1):30–4.
23. Sudak DM, Goldberg DA. Trends in psychotherapy training: A national survey of psychiatry residency training. Acad Psychiatry 2012;36(5):369–73.
24. Calabrese C, Sciolla A, Zisook S, et al. Psychiatric residents' views of quality of psychotherapy training and psychotherapy competencies: a multisite survey. Acad Psychiatry 2010;34(1):13–20.
25. Sudak DM, Beck JS, Wright J. Cognitive behavioral therapy: a blueprint for attaining and assessing psychiatry resident competency. Acad Psychiatry 2003;27(3):154–9.
26. Weerasekera P. The state of psychotherapy supervision: recommendations for future training. Int Rev Psychiatry 2013;25(3):255–64.
27. Pagano J, Kyle BN, Johnson TL. A Manual by Any Other Name: Identifying Psychotherapy Manuals for Resident Training. Acad Psychiatry 2017;41(1):44–50.
28. Weissman MM, Sanderson WC. Promises and problems in modern psychotherapy: The need for increased training in evidence-based treatments. In: Hager Med. Modern psychiatry: Challenges in educating health professionals to meet new needs. 2002:132–65.
29. Shedler J. Where is the Evidence for "Evidence-Based" Therapy? Psychiatr Clin 2018;41(2):319–29.
30. Binder JL. Key competencies in brief dynamic psychotherapy: clinical practice beyond the manual. New York: Guilford press; 2004.
31. Steinert C, Munder T, Rabung S, et al. Psychodynamic therapy: as efficacious as other empirically supported treatments? A meta-analysis testing equivalence of outcomes. Am J Psychiatry 2017;174(10):943–53.
32. Shedler J. The efficacy of psychodynamic psychotherapy. Am Psychol 2010;65(2):98.
33. Gabbard GO. Preserving the person in contemporary psychiatry. Psychiatr Clin 2018;41(2):183–91.
34. Gastelum ED, Hyun AM, Goldberg DA, et al. Is that an unconscious fantasy or an automatic thought? Challenges of learning multiple psychotherapies simultaneously. J Am Acad Psychoanal Dyn Psychiatr 2011;39(1):111–32.
35. Feinstein R, Heiman N, Yager J. Common factors affecting psychotherapy outcomes: Some implications for teaching psychotherapy. J Psychiatr Practice® 2015;21(3):180–9.
36. Weerasekera P, Antony MM, Bellissimo A, et al. Competency assessment in the McMaster psychotherapy program. Acad Psychiatry 2003;27(3):166–73.
37. Plakun EM, Sudak DM, Goldberg D. The Y model: an integrated, evidence-based approach to teaching psychotherapy competencies. J Psychiatr Practice® 2009;15(1):5–11.
38. Cabaniss DL, Holoshitz Y. Different patients, different therapies: optimizing treatment using differential psychotherapuetics. New York: WW Norton & Company; 2019.
39. Feinstein RE, Yager J. Advanced psychotherapy training: Psychotherapy Scholars' Track, and the apprenticeship model. Acad Psychiatry 2013;37(4):248–53.

40. Cabaniss DL, Arbuckle MR. Course and lab: a new model for supervision. Journal Academic Psychiatry 2011.
41. Barnett JE. Utilizing technological innovations to enhance psychotherapy supervision, training, and outcomes. Psychotherapy 2011;48(2):103.
42. Manring J, Greenberg RP, Gregory R, et al. Learning psychotherapy in the digital age. Psychotherapy 2011;48(2):119.
43. DeRoma VM, Hickey DA, Stanek KM. Methods of supervision in marriage and family therapist training: a brief report. North Am J Psychol 2007;9(3).
44. Weerasekera P. Psychotherapy update for the practicing psychiatrist: promoting evidence-based practice. Focus 2010;8(1):3–18.
45. Ravitz P, Silver I. Advances in psychotherapy education. Can J Psychiatry 2004; 49(4):230–7.
46. Winer JA, Klamen DL. Psychotherapy Supervision. Acad Psychiatry 1997;21(3): 141–7.
47. Bender E. Gabbard explains dos and don'ts of teaching psychotherapy. Psychiatr News 2005;30. Accessed April 15.
48. Peters GA, Cormier LS, Cormier WH. Effects of modeling, rehearsal, feedback, and remediation on acquisition of a counseling strategy. J Couns Psychol 1978;25(3):231.

Competency-Based Assessment in Psychiatric Education: A Systems Approach

John Q. Young, MD, MPP, PhD[a],*, Eric S. Holmboe, MD[b],
Jason R. Frank, MD, MA(Ed), FRCPC[c,d]

KEYWORDS

- Competency-based medical education • Competency-based assessment
- Workplace-based assessment • Psychiatry • Programmatic assessment • Validity
- Medical education • System

KEY POINTS

- Medical education programs are failing to meet the health needs of patients and communities. Misalignments exist on multiple levels, including content (what trainees learn), pedagogy (how trainees learn), and culture (why trainees learn).
- Competency-based medical education has emerged in response to these shortcomings.
- These efforts will not succeed unless competency-based assessment programs are designed to simultaneously produce lifelong learners who can self-regulate their own growth as well as trustworthy processes that determine and accelerate readiness for independent practice.
- The key to effectively doing so is situating assessment within a carefully designed system with several, critical, interacting components: workplace-based assessment, ongoing faculty development, learning analytics, longitudinal coaching, and fit-for-purpose clinical competency committees.

BACKGROUND
Emergence of Outcomes-Based Education

Over the past two plus decades, numerous national and international reports have found critical deficiencies in medical education, including psychiatric medical

Funding: J.Q. Young, ABPN Research Award (2019–2020).
[a] Department of Psychiatry, Donald and Barbara Zucker School of Medicine at Hofstra/Northwell and the Zucker Hillside Hospital at Northwell Health, Glen Oaks, NY, USA; [b] Accreditation Council for Graduate Medical Education, 401 North Michigan Avenue, Chicago, IL 60611, USA; [c] Royal College of Physicians and Surgeons of Canada, 774 Echo Drive, Ottawa, Ontario K15 5NB, Canada; [d] Education, Department of Emergency Medicine, University of Ottawa, Ottawa, Ontario, Canada
* Corresponding author. Zucker Hillside Hospital, 75-59 263rd Street, Kaufman Building, Glen Oaks, NY 11004,
E-mail address: Jyoung9@northwell.edu

education (PsyME). These deficiencies include suboptimal patient outcomes, unacceptable variability in the abilities of trainees upon graduation, poor alignment between what trainees learn and the competencies required to provide safe and effective care in the twenty-first century healthcare systems, and a significant gap between evidence based instructional technique and actual practice in medical education.[1-4] These and other reports have called for fundamental and far reaching reforms.[5,6] In an effort to better align the medical education continuum with population health needs, regulatory bodies developed a new approach in the mid to late 1990s.[7] Accreditation bodies shifted focus from structure and process measures (eg, time-based rotations) to educational outcomes.[8-10] For example, in 2001, the Accreditation Council for Graduate Medical Education (ACGME) recommended that graduation from residency become contingent on demonstrated competence in the now-familiar 6 core domains. Similar reforms took place in other countries, such as in Canada and The Netherlands (the CanMEDS framework) and the United Kingdom (Tomorrow's Doctors).[11] Since then, programs in the United States have been required to base promotion decisions on demonstrated competence in the 6 core domains.[7]

In this context, competency-based medical education (CBME) emerged as an outcomes-based approach to the design, implementation, assessment, and evaluation of medical education programs.[10] The approach is fundamentally oriented to outcomes; that is, the abilities of graduates. In CBME, the outcomes or competencies are derived from an analysis of societal and patient needs; that is, the abilities that physicians need on graduation in order to meet population needs and effectively function in the emerging health care delivery systems. CBME then works backward to design and implement curricula against these competencies.[12] CBME emphasizes instructional techniques that are learner specific, flexible, and time variable. More recently, with the recognition of burnout and the devastating effects it can have on skill acquisition, CBME has recognized the importance of learning cultures and processes that promote resilience and well-being.[13]

Reforms to Better Align Psychiatric Medical Education with Population Health

The emergence of outcomes-based education has stimulated efforts to realign systems of medical education with patient and societal needs.[14,15] These efforts have addressed misalignment on several levels, including content (what people learn), pedagogy (how people learn), and culture (why people learn). There is reform in content. Curricula are evolving to prepare graduates to practice in delivery systems that use team-based, population-oriented, technology-enabled care for the longitudinal management of chronic disease rather than individual-based, episodic management of acute illness.[14,16] In psychiatry, this has included the inclusion of courses and rotations dedicated to learning integrated care, tele-psychiatry, clinical neuroscience, system approaches to quality improvement and patient safety, and evidence-based pharmacotherapy and psychotherapies.[17-22] Moreover, there is reform in pedagogy. Instructional techniques are increasingly using evidence-based strategies to more effectively integrate formal knowledge and clinical experience, develop habits of inquiry and improvement, and support the formation of professional identities.[15,18,23] In addition, in the face of endemic burnout, there is reform in culture and a return to the "why" of medicine. Education is beginning to address how to change learning environments and cultures in order to foster resilience and enduring engagement rather than burnout.[24-26]

Key Enabler of Reform: Competency-Based Assessment

These movements all offer hope that the disconnects and misalignments between medical education and health system and patient needs may be addressed. However, these efforts will ultimately not succeed unless 2 fundamental challenges are met. First, psychiatric medical education (PsyME) must learn how to produce lifelong learners who can self-regulate their own learning by continually incorporating the exponentially increasing volume and complexity of new evidence into their practice of medicine. Otherwise, it will not be possible to close the quality chasm that exists between actual care and best care, and our future physicians will not adapt to their new roles in emerging care delivery models. Current medical education programs produce physicians who are unable to adequately learn (i.e., change their practice patterns) once they enter independent practice. For example, roughly half the care provided in the United States across specialties is not consistent with evidence-based practice.[27] In addition, the time lag for physicians to adopt newly proven effective practices is nearly 2 decades, and may be even longer for physicians to "deadopt" practices subsequently shown to be ineffective.[28–30]

Second, PsyME must learn how to gather and interpret robust performance data so that competency acquisition is accelerated and residents graduate only if and when they are ready for independent practice; that is, when they possess the competencies required to provide safe, person-centered, and effective care to patients and communities within health systems. Otherwise, there will be no data to drive continuous quality improvement of curricula and learning environments, support time-variable training, and ensure alignment between medical education and health care systems.

Meeting these 2 challenges requires the capacity to capture meaningful educational outcomes in a system of assessment that supports self-regulated learning and competence as well as trustworthy decisions about readiness for practice.[31] This requirement has led to substantial and sustained efforts internationally to develop effective ways to assess these competencies.

Implementation Challenges with Competency-Based Assessment

However, implementation of CBME has encountered significant challenges. Some have argued that the units of assessment (eg, milestones and competencies) are too numerous and/or too abstract for educators to meaningfully evaluate.[32,33]

In addition, traditional methods of assessment, which focus on "knows" and "knows how," have been insufficient to assess competence in the workplace; that is, what doctors actually do in practice.[34–37] This situation has led to the development of workplace-based assessment (WBA), a topic explored in detail in a companion review article. In short, although WBA strategies (eg, direct observation tools, multisource feedback) have been developed, many have been plagued by validity concerns.[38,39] For example, faculty members often do not use the same frame of reference when completing a WBA and their feedback often lacks meaningfulness for the learner, leading to trivialization.[31] Research findings indicate that narrative comments provide helpful guidance to learners and enhance summative decisions, especially when combined with quantitative ratings.[40–42] However, the narrative comments are also plagued by variable quality and the purposeful use of vague or coded language that can be difficult for the both the learner and the clinical competency committee to interpret.[43,44]

Moreover, WBA efforts have not adequately engaged the learner as a coproducer,[45] a critical feature if systems are to generate physicians who are motivated[46] and able to regulate their own learning.[47] The provision of high-quality external data is necessary, but not sufficient, for self-directed learning.[48,49] Self-directed learning requires considerable external direction and scaffolding.[50] Coaching has been shown to increase residents' abilities to recognize and reflect on learning opportunities as well as seek additional activities to improve performance.[51] The creation of a psychologically safe, interpersonal space in which so-called imposter syndrome and other doubts can be addressed will help trainees and their faculty and coaches move from a fixed to a growth mindset and become more resilient within environments that expose their inadequate skills.[52]

In addition, even when assessment tools with evidence for validity have been implemented in a way that engages the learner, the assessment activity generally is not part of a system of assessment that is aligned with the curriculum and that combines multiple assessments and components into a process that supports high-quality feedback and trustworthy summative decisions by clinical competency committees (CCCs).[36,38]

COMPETENCY-BASED ASSESSMENT IN PSYCHIATRIC MEDICAL EDUCATION

To address these challenges effectively, competency-based assessment (CBA) for PsyME must simultaneously optimize 3 goals: (1) maximal learning through formative assessment (assessment for learning); (2) robust high-stakes decision making (eg, promotion or selection) through summative assessment (assessment of learning); and (3) ongoing improvements in the curriculum through programmatic assessment.[31] The remainder of this article focuses primarily on the first 2 goals. As such, the CBA system must promote both self-regulated growth and clinical competence as judged by a trustworthy process. These purposes must be held together. The key to effectively doing so is situating these activities within a carefully designed system of assessment.

System of Assessment

One of the most important insights to emerge from the early efforts to implement CBA is the understanding that the validity and, ultimately, the effectiveness of CBA are not primarily about the assessment tools but about how the various assessment activities interact with each other and relate to the overall goals. This insight has led to a shift in

Table 1
Design principles for a system of competency-based assessment

Design Principle	Brief Description
(1) Coherent	Individual assessments are coordinated and aligned around the same purposes within a common framework
(2) Continuous	Assessments are ongoing, frequent, and embedded throughout the curriculum
(3) Comprehensive	Each competency is assessed multiple times by several methods; the assessment activities, taken together, serve formative, summative, and programmatic assessment
(4) Feasible	The components of the system of assessment are practical, sensible, and doable for the given stakeholders, context, and purposes
(5) Purpose driven	The CBA system supports the purposes for which it was created, including robust formative, summative, and programmatic assessment
(6) Acceptable	The CBA system is credible and acceptable to the stakeholders, including the learners, staff, patients, faculty, school or institution, and regulatory bodies
(7) Transparent and equitable	The ownership, access, and use of the assessment data is clear to all stakeholders; systematic steps are taken to detect and minimize bias and promote fair outcomes

Data from Norcini J, Anderson MB, Bollela V, et al. 2018 Consensus framework for good assessment. Med Teach. 2018:1-8.

focus from the psychometric properties of assessment tools to the design of the assessment system.[38,53,54] In 2018, an international group of educational researchers and thought leaders published a consensus framework for a good system of assessment. The good system has the following features[38]: (1) coherent; (2) continuous; (3) comprehensive; (4) feasible; (5) purpose driven; (6) acceptable; and (7) transparent and equitable (**Table 1**).

The good-enough CBA system operationalizes these design principles and blends multiple assessments to achieve different purposes (eg, formative and summative) for a variety of stakeholders (eg, patients, residents, faculty, CCCs, regulators). This system includes the use of assessment instruments with evidence for validity but also protected spaces for the assessment activities (eg, direct observation and structured feedback), engaged and activated faculty and learners who are oriented to a similar conception of the performance dimensions, and a culture that values growth.

To operationalize these principles, the good-enough CBA system has several interacting components: WBA, ongoing faculty development, learning analytics, longitudinal coaching, and trustworthy clinical competence decision-making processes (**Fig. 1**). Each of these components is reviewed here.

Workplace-Based Assessment

WBAs are at the center of a CBA system (for a detailed examination of WBA, please see the companion article "Advancing Workplace-based Assessment in Psychiatric Education," in this issue).[55] WBAs focus on what trainees actually do with patients and team members and this forms the basis for identifying growth edges and determining readiness for independent practice. WBAs typically serve both formative purposes (ie, feedback in the moment for the purpose of growth) and summative purposes (ie, aggregated data to inform promotion and advancement decisions).

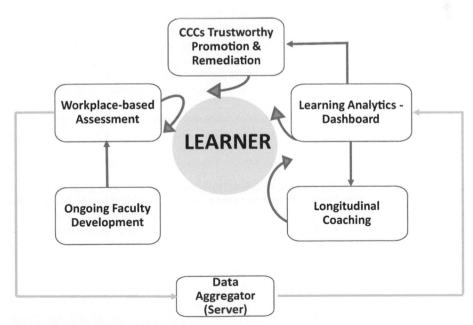

Fig. 1. Components of a CBA system.

In developing the WBAs, PsyME programs must first choose the framework for assessment. PsyME programs should also use multiple types of WBAs, each administered multiple times with multiple assessors.[31] The use of multiples helps overcome important sources of bias. Multiple methods help to compensate for the limitations of any 1 technique. Multiple assessments of a given competency or entrustable professional activity (EPA) help overcome so-called one-offs (eg, the resident was preoccupied by a personal matter that interfered with performance during one assessment) and to develop a more stable and complete view of a trainee's skill. Multiple and diverse assessors compensate for the biases (eg, halo effects, leniency, gender, race, sexual orientation etc...) that influence any given faculty member's judgment.

The most common WBA tools include multisource feedback (MSF) from patients, staff, and/or peers, chart-stimulated recall, direct observation, end-rotation global feedback, portfolios, and practice-based audit. Several psychiatry specific tools have been published. Multisource feedback programs for psychiatry trainees have been implemented with evidence for feasibility and validity.[56] The Psychopharmacotherapy-structured Clinical Observation (P-SCO) is a direct observation and feedback tool designed to assess the EPA of a follow-up visit.[57–60] Similarly, evidence for validity has also been developed for the EPA of a psychiatric diagnostic interview.[61] Some psychiatry programs have implemented EPAs, most commonly in the end-rotation global assessment.[62,63]

Ongoing Faculty Development

Although the WBA tools should be developed and adapted according to validity principles, validity resides more in the users of the instrument than in the instruments that are used.[31] Faculty possess idiosyncratic frames of reference and often provide vague narrative feedback,[43] which undermines the validity of the information for summative decisions and the utility of the information for growth. Faculty and resident training are essential and must address multiple skill sets:

1. Direct observation of trainees while supporting their autonomy.
2. A shared mental model of the performance dimensions (ie, for a given EPA or competency, what are the key components, in behavioral terms, that must occur in order to meet the standard for independent practice?) and the frame of reference (ie, are you rating the resident compared with peers or an external standard?).
3. Crafting quality narrative comments.[64,65]
4. Feedback as a bidirectional dialogue, sometimes called coaching in the moment, that collaboratively constructs a shared assessment and then generates a specific plan for action with follow-up.[66] This model is a significant departure from the traditional unidirectional flow of feedback from the expert to the trainee.

To be effective, training must be frequent, multimodal, multitouch, and longitudinal and incorporate a broad range of educational strategies, including larger-scale workshops, more frequent service-specific trainings, online video modules, near peer support, and simulation with standardized learners. Residents and faculty need to be trained in how to coproduce learning and clinical care; that is, how to seek and engage with feedback in clinical contexts, a set of skills that is often neglected.[36] The ACGME's Regional Faculty Development Workshops for CBA are an excellent model.[67,68] Intensive faculty development ensures that each data point is maximally informative to the learner: information rich, expressed in verbal and written formats, and engaged within a supervisory relationship focused on growth. Finally, residency programs should look to create longitudinal supervisory relationships in which a strong educational alliance can develop and support honest and productive growth conversations.

Learning Analytics and Data Visualization

The thoughtful implementation of WBA tools into direct observation and structured feedback programs supported by ongoing faculty and resident training help to ensure that each assessment given to a trainee is maximally rich. Variance will exist. Two faculty may rate the same resident encounter with a patient differently. These differences can arise for multiple reasons. Each faculty may value 2 different, equally important components of the task. One attending may focus on the screening for adverse effects, substance use, and suicide risk and overlook other important competencies, whereas the other may focus on how the trainee establishes an alliance and elicits the narrative. The variance in this case enhances the quality of the feedback. In contrast, one faculty may see the provision of supportive techniques during a medication visit as inappropriate, whereas the other does not. This kind of variance may reflect contradictory notions of the task and is unwarranted.

Thus, although some of the variance will be meaningful and important to embrace, some will also arise from bias (eg, selective abstraction, gender, race, premature judgment, idiosyncratic beliefs etc...). All of this points to the fact that any single assessment is limited by content specificity; that is, that individual performance is context dependent (eg, specific day, time, patient, attending, diagnosis, emotional state).[69,70] There are several key strategies to manage this challenge in addition to a robust program of ongoing faculty development. First, to capture a stable and trustworthy picture of a trainee's performance, multiple data points need to be aggregated across multiple assessors and contexts.[71] The number of data points should increase with the stakes of the assessment decision.[31] Second, PsyME needs to incorporate advanced learner analytics when aggregating data. These tools can be used to identify patterns of skew in the assessment system that may reflect unwanted bias (eg, gender, race, rotation sequence, assessor, etc...). The detected bias can inform faculty development and coaching efforts. In addition, the analytics can manage the bias by generating risk-adjusted performance propensity curves for each learner that account for factors such as rotation order, specific attendings assigned, race, gender, and so forth.[72] Third, natural language processors will soon be available to help capture themes from the large amounts of narrative data that a good-enough CBA system should generate. This tool will be enormously helpful to coaches and CCCs alike.

In addition, the quantitative and narrative data need to be visualized in dashboards. A dashboard offers a platform for high-level data display, combined with drill-down options for more detail on quantitative and qualitative measures of learner performance. This information, combined with display of metrics indicating expected levels of performance, supports summative judgment and also enables evidence-informed feedback discussions between residents and their faculty advisors or coaches to inform robust learning planning. With advanced learning analytics, dashboards can support both self-regulated learning and summative decisions with, for example, control charts that depict the competency acquisition trajectories for each individual trainee, including when change is meaningful versus noise.[73,74] Data visualization in the form of dashboards combined with learning analytics is critical to avoid cognitive overload and support proper interpretation. Dashboard design needs to be carefully aligned with the needs of the end user. The design may be different for coaching versus clinical competency committee uses. Moreover, the needs of the end user change and evolve; it is important to have the built-in capability to constantly revise and customize dashboards on an ongoing basis.[72]

The most powerful use of learning analytics centers on the aggregation and analysis of large amounts of data in order to depict, perhaps via risk-adjusted performance propensity curves, where a trainee's skill level is relative to the stage of training and readiness for independent practice. These sorts of tools empower trainees, coaches, and CCCs for both self-regulated growth and for trustworthy promotion decisions.

Learning analytics also has tremendous possibilities for trainees who are having difficulties. For example, advanced learning analytics within a CBA system enables earlier identification and, just as importantly, provision of support to underperforming trainees.[75] In recently published data, researchers examined a longitudinal cohort of emergency medicine, family medicine, and internal medicine residents over their entire residency programs.[76] The analysis showed that a milestone rating of lower than level 2.5 at the end of the second year (of the 3-year programs) had a predictive probability of not attaining level 4 for that subcompetency ranging from 15% to 67%, depending on the program and the subcompetency. In data not yet published, a large internal medicine program has been able to use advanced analytics of direct observation data to identify within 6 months of beginning residency which trainees are at risk for not meeting program expectations.[77] These analytical techniques, as they are further developed and adopted, can improve the recognition and management of learning challenges and ultimately reduce the probability of graduates possessing key skill deficiencies.

Suffice it to say, advanced learning analytics has much to offer. This kind of sophistication, with the capability to manage skew and potential bias, aggregate and analyze large amounts of data, and deliver in formats that support catalytic growth and summative decision making, will be critical if time-variable training is to be actualized. If done correctly, the tools give CCCs much more confidence in making judgments about readiness for independent practice. However, even with these techniques, the quality of the output depends on the quality of the input. The adage "garbage, in, garbage out" still holds. To add value, analytics must be incorporated into a system of assessment that captures high-quality data. Hence, the importance of the underlying program of WBA, including the tools, faculty development, and learning cultures.

Longitudinal Coaching

Providing feedback, even if purely formative, is not enough to stimulate growth. Learners must review, reflect, discuss, and apply the feedback.[45,78–80] However, medical students and residents typically do not engage in self-regulated learning (ie, engage in reflection and self-improvement on their own accord), a finding seen in both formative and summative assessment.[81,82] Studies in PsyME have had similar findings. For example, although residents in one psychiatry program uniformly appreciated the specific feedback provided to them via WBA tools, they rarely returned to the feedback after initial receipt.[48,83] This finding is concerning and represents a significant threat to the impact on learning and, ultimately, the validity of a CBA program, if one of the primary purposes is to graduate lifelong learners. It has become increasingly clear that trainees, in addition to high-quality external data, need assistance with self-assessment and growth. One possible solution is to provide trainees with a coach who stands apart from the 2 assessment processes described so far, feedback in the moment, and higher-stakes advancement decisions. If coaching relationships are longitudinal, there may be a better opportunity to develop the psychological safety and interpersonal comfort necessary for conversations that touch on information that is potentially identity-threatening or inconsistent with self-assessment.[45,78]

Programs in PsyME need to develop and implement evidence-based coaching programs. Longitudinal coaches need to be selected and trained to create a safe place in

Step	Action
Table 2 **Longitudinal coaching: typical action and reflection cycles**	
1	The coach and learner (dyad) build through conversation a shared understanding of the standards of performance
2	The dyad reflect on performance by reviewing dashboards containing both quantitative and narrative data
3	The dyad create individual learning objectives, identify opportunities for deliberate practice[87] of the independent learning objectives, and aggregate these objectives into action plans
4	The resident shares action plans with supervising residents and attendings to coconstruct practice during daily work
5	The coach and resident, at a subsequent meeting, close the loop on prior action plans and review new data to understand the quality of changes that took place and begin the next learning cycle

which trainees can learn how to identify growth edges and set action plans. Such programs should be grounded in positive psychology; foster self-regulated learning[84]; use a bidirectional, constructivist feedback model[85]; and promote a growth mindset and work toward a personal best.[86] Residents and coaches should embrace a coproduction model[45] to develop residents as learners with agency. This kind of coaching program will entail a predictable cycle of reflection and action (deliberate practice[87]) **(Table 2)**.

The longitudinal coaching relationship can start after the match, even before matriculation. The initial work should focus on benchmarking the initial skillset with respect to both clinical and self-regulated growth abilities. Benchmarking can be supported with the use of standardized patient simulations during orientation. Moreover, coaches need to continuously reorient residents and themselves to the purpose of this work, namely to encourage and support resident well-being while they engage in iterative, vigorous performance improvement. In addition, to help develop the resident's intrinsic motivation, the coach will want to support the resident's autonomy, competence, and self-efficacy.[88,89]

Future work in PsyME should prioritize developing model coaching programs with training materials. The potential benefits of this kind of coaching program are significant, especially if they can generate residents skilled in self-regulated learning who are, therefore, more engaged in their work and less vulnerable to burnout. Resident receptivity will be facilitated through reflection on feedback that is perceived as credible (ie, meaningful) and in the context of a longitudinal relationship so that the feedback is perceived as intended to support.[90,91] Again, although the provision of high-quality feedback data with advanced analytics is not sufficient for a CBA system, a coaching program without high-quality and rigorous data will be severely limited.

Reengineered Clinical Competency or Advancement Committees

The CCCs or their analogs in undergraduate medical education (hereafter simply referred to as CCCs) should have the same 2 purposes as the overall CBA system: trustworthy judgments about readiness for independent practice (public accountability) and ongoing guidance to learners to support their growth (including remediation). The CCC serves these purposes through the synthesis of multiple quantitative and qualitative assessments. **Fig. 2** highlights the several aspects of a high-

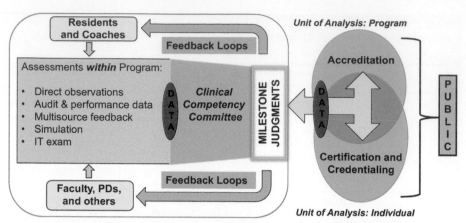

Fig. 2. Clinical competency committee: data synthesizer. IT, information technology; PDs, program directors. (*Adapted from* The Milestones Guidebook, with permission.)

performing CCC, including a combination of multiple assessment methods and assessors, learners as active agents and coconstructors of assessment, and the program's accountability to the public.

Most CCCs fall far short of **Fig. 2**. A 2015 study of 34 program directors at 5 institutions discovered that most CCCs relied on global, end-of-rotation evaluations rather than using programmatic assessment with multiple tools and data points, focused on problem residents more than they spent time discussing typical residents, and lacked faculty development or training for CCC members.[92]

Despite these challenges, the evidence base for CCCs is rapidly evolving and provides important guidance on how CCCs can better meet their mandate.[93] **Table 3** highlights key recommendations from this literature. One set of recommendations centers on CCC members. To improve the quality and defensibility of CCCs' judgments, CCC members should possess a growth mindset. This mindset is critical if

Table 3
Key features of fit-for-purpose clinical competency committees

Feature	Characteristics
Members	Growth mindset Shared mental model of progression Diverse and inclusive
Process	Triangulation across multiple data points from multiple sources Deliberation proportional to the clarity of the information Explicit management of bias Transparency to key stakeholders
Decision support	Software that aggregate and visualize all data points and identify meaningful change Learning analytics that identify possible meaningful change (negative or positive)
Actions	Early recognition of when a trainee is off trajectory Remediation/growth plans that are highly specific to the individual

they are to rebalance toward formative assessment and shift the focus from problem identification toward a developmental approach that benefits all learners. CCC members must also possess a shared mental model of progression and what constitutes competence for each EPA or milestone. CCC members should also be diverse and trained in health equity, inclusion, and bias. Emerging data suggest that bias affects both numerical and quantitative data. Performance ratings have been shown to be systematically lower for women and under-represented minorities.[94,95] Narrative data have been shown to reinforce stereotypes.[96] Programs must engage in authentic and explicit discussion and training to reduce implicit and explicit bias.

Another set of recommendations focus on the decision-making processes. CCC members should be trained to review the assessment data ahead of the meeting but to not come to the CCC meeting with a decision already determined. There should be a consistent and structured process. The process itself can look different depending on the program. Some CCCs assign learners to specific members and ask the latter to present a summary. Alternatively, some programs have each resident presented in a debatelike format. Mentors present the residents accomplishments and a second reviewer presents challenges.[97] Visual aids and dashboards are crucial to aid interpretation, help focus the discussion, and facilitate recognition of when a trainee is off trajectory. Hierarchy can suppress dissent. CCCs should always start with the person most at risk in the hierarchical chain. Effective group process leads to better decisions than those made by individuals and to identification of problems otherwise overlooked.[98] The group process should use methods demonstrated to improve trustworthiness, such as triangulation across multiple data points from multiple sources, management of bias, and deliberation proportional to the clarity of information. Current research is focused on best practices for CCC decision making when lacking adequate data.[99]

CCCs that use high-quality data and deliberative processes generate highly personalized growth plans and trustworthy summative decisions, creating the future basis for time-variable training.[54,92,100,101]

EVALUATING THE COMPETENCY-BASED ASSESSMENT SYSTEM

An important future question centers on how the effectiveness of CBA systems in PsyME is evaluated. Such an evaluation must account for the components interacting both with each other as well as with varied and unpredictable clinical and educational contexts. For interventions that occur in a complex adaptive system, implementation science frameworks that account for this complexity may be the most suitable evaluation design.[102] This kind of approach leads to evaluation at 3 levels: (1) individual components, (2) component interactions (how components relate to each other and the whole), and (3) overall system performance (clinical performance of the trainees and their dispositions toward growth).[103] For individual components, evaluation can focus on fidelity to the particular model of WBA, faculty development, longitudinal coaching, and so forth. Surveys, focus groups, and direct observation of processes (eg, video/audio tape of feedback, coaching sessions, or CCCs) can assess quality against these indicators and probe barriers.

To understand how individual components interact and function together, 2 strategies seem relevant. First, the evaluation can focus on the experience of the end-users (ie, the trainees, faculty, and the CCCs). For trainees, this might include data such as the number and quality of direct observations, completed WBAs, coaching sessions, and action plans. For faculty, this might include the ease of use of the WBAs, the impact of the WBAs on their relationship with trainees, and the number and quality of completed WBAs. For CCCs, this might include data that characterize the quality and amount of information provided for their decisions. Second, implementation science frameworks such as the Consolidated Framework for Implementation Research can be used to identify factors that influence residents' and CCCs' perceptions of credibility and utility.[102]

To evaluate overall performance of the CBA system, measures should focus on the overall intended outcomes (ie, self-regulated learning and clinical competence). Toward that end, residents could complete measures that assess dispositions toward learning and growth, including self-regulated learning, motivation, curiosity, resilience, burnout, and aspiration for excellence. Clinical performance measures could include time to attainment of milestone and/or EPA competencies, patient experience ratings, other MSF data, resident-sensitive quality measures, and postgraduation performance (fellowship milestone data and survey data from employers).

SUMMARY

Medical education, including PsyME, has come under scrutiny for key deficiencies, including suboptimal patient outcomes in health care systems, unacceptable variability in the abilities of graduates after medical training, poor alignment between what trainees learn and the competencies required to provide safe and effective care in the emerging twenty-first century care delivery systems, and a significant gap between evidence-based instructional technique and actual practice in medical education. Recent recognition of endemic burnout as an adverse effect of medical education programs and culture have added additional pressure for reform. At the same time, CBME in general, and CBA in particular, has emerged. Medical education programs have responded with promising innovations in content, pedagogy, and culture. These changes offer hope. However, the ability to deliver on the promise of these innovations lies in developing CBA for PsyME that simultaneously optimizes 3 goals: (1) maximal learning through formative assessment and coaching (assessment for learning); (2) robust and trustworthy high-stakes decision making (eg, promotion or selection) through summative assessment (assessment of learning); and (3) ongoing improvements in the curriculum through programmatic assessment. The key to effectively doing so is designing a system of CBA with several critical components: WBA, ongoing faculty development, learning analytics, longitudinal coaching, and fit-for-purpose CCCs. Implementation will encounter significant challenges; however, the evidence base is rapidly expanding, as are practical guidebooks.[104] Successful implementation holds great promise. PsyME will be much better positioned to promote both self-regulated growth and clinical competence and, with trustworthy and rigorous educational outcomes, to argue for increased flexibility in curricular innovation and even time-variable training.

CLINICAL PEARLS FOR COMPETENCY-BASED ASSESSMENT IN PSYCHIATRIC EDUCATION: A SYSTEMS APPROACH

- CBA should simultaneously promote self-regulated growth and trustworthy judgments about readiness for independent practice.
- Assessment activities must be situated within a system of assessment.
- Key components of a system of assessment include WBA, ongoing faculty development, learning analytics, longitudinal coaching, and fit-for-purpose CCCs.

CLINICAL PEARLS FOR ADVANCING WORKPLACE-BASED ASSESSMENT IN PSYCHIATRIC EDUCATION: KEY DESIGN AND IMPLEMENTATION ISSUES

- WBA shifts the focus from knows and knows how to what the trainee actually does with patients and team members in the workplace.
- WBAs generate information to support assessment of learning and assessment for learning.
- High-quality WBAs require alignment with the curriculum, evidence for validity, a coherent framework, and suitable platforms.
- Threats to validity include poor instrument design, inadequate opportunities for direct observation, inter-rater variability, and cultures and practices that prize achievement more than growth.

DISCLOSURES

Funding: John Q. Young, MD, MPP, PhD - ABPN Research Award (2019-2020).

REFERENCES

1. Frenk J, Chen L, Bhutta ZA, et al. Health professionals for a new century: transforming education to strengthen health systems in an interdependent world. Lancet 2010;376(9756):1923–58.
2. Lucey CR. Medical education: part of the problem and part of the solution. JAMA Intern Med 2013;173(17):1639–43.
3. Cooke M, Irby DM, O'Brien BC, Carnegie Foundation for the Advancement of Teaching. Educating physicians : a call for reform of medical school and residency. 1st edition. San Francisco (CA): Jossey-Bass; 2010.
4. Eden J, Berwick DM, Wilensky GR, Institute of Medicine (U.S.). Committee on the Governance and Financing of Graduate Medical Education. Graduate medical education that meets the nation's health needs. Washington, DC: The National Academies Press; 2014.
5. Thibault GE. Reforming health professions education will require culture change and closer ties between classroom and practice. Health Aff (Millwood) 2013;32(11):1928–32.
6. Skochelak SE. A decade of reports calling for change in medical education: what do they say? Acad Med 2010;85(9 Suppl):S26–33.
7. Nasca TJ, Philibert I, Brigham T, et al. The next GME accreditation system–rationale and benefits. N Engl J Med 2012;366(11):1051–6.
8. Carraccio C, Wolfsthal SD, Englander R, et al. Shifting paradigms: from Flexner to competencies. Acad Med 2002;77(5):361–7.
9. Leach DC. A model for GME: shifting from process to outcomes. A progress report from the accreditation council for graduate medical education. Med Educ 2004;38(1):12–4.
10. Frank JR, Snell LS, Cate OT, et al. Competency-based medical education: theory to practice. Med Teach 2010;32(8):638–45.
11. Frank JR, Danoff D. The CanMEDS initiative: implementing an outcomes-based framework of physician competencies. Med Teach 2007;29(7):642–7.
12. Frank JR, Mungroo R, Ahmad Y, et al. Toward a definition of competency-based education in medicine: a systematic review of published definitions. Med Teach 2010;32(8):631–7.

13. Dauphinee WD. Building a core competency assessment program for all stake-holders: the design and building of sailing ships can inform core competency frameworks. Adv Health Sci Educ Theory Pract 2020;25(1):189–93.
14. Frenk J, Chen L, Bhutta ZA, et al. Health professionals for a new century: transforming education to strengthen health systems in an interdependent world. Lancet 2010;376(9756):1923–58.
15. Cooke M, Irby DM, O'Brien BC. Carnegie foundation for the advancement of teaching. Educating physicians : a call for reform of medical school and residency. 1st edition. San Francisco (CA): Jossey-Bass; 2010.
16. Lucey CR. Medical education: part of the problem and part of the solution. JAMA Intern Med 2013;173(17):1639–43.
17. Arbuckle MR, Weinberg M, Cabaniss DL, et al. Training psychiatry residents in quality improvement: an integrated, year-long curriculum. Acad Psychiatry 2013;37(1):42–5.
18. Arbuckle MR, Travis MJ, Eisen J, et al. Transforming psychiatry from the classroom to the clinic: lessons from the national neuroscience curriculum initiative. Acad Psychiatry 2020;44(1):29–36.
19. Patel E, Muthusamy V, Young JQ. Delivering on the promise of CLER: a patient safety rotation that aligns resident education with hospital processes. Acad Med 2018;93(6):898–903.
20. Sunderji N, Ion A, Huynh D, et al. Advancing integrated care through psychiatric workforce development: a systematic review of educational interventions to train psychiatrists in integrated care. Can J Psychiatry 2018;63(8):513–25.
21. Crawford A, Sunderji N, Lopez J, et al. Defining competencies for the practice of telepsychiatry through an assessment of resident learning needs. BMC Med Educ 2016;16:28.
22. Hilty D, Chan S, Torous J, et al. A Framework for competencies for the use of mobile technologies in psychiatry and medicine: scoping review. JMIR Mhealth Uhealth 2020;8(2):e12229.
23. Young JQ, Sugarman R, Schwartz J, et al. Exploring residents' experience of career development scholarship tracks: a qualitative case study using social cognitive career theory. Teach Learn Med 2020;32(5):522–30.
24. Shanafelt TD, Dyrbye LN, West CP. Addressing physician burnout: the way forward. JAMA 2017;317(9):901–2.
25. Goldman ML, Bernstein CA, Konopasek L, et al. An intervention framework for institutions to meet new ACGME common program requirements for physician well-being. Acad Psychiatry 2018;42(4):542–7.
26. Young JQ, Schwartz J, Thakker K, et al. Where passion meets need: a longitudinal, self-directed program to help residents discover meaning and develop as scholars. Acad Psychiatry 2020;44(4):455–60.
27. McGlynn EA, Asch SM, Adams J, et al. The quality of health care delivered to adults in the United States. N Engl J Med 2003;348(26):2635–45.
28. Morris ZS, Wooding S, Grant J. The answer is 17 years, what is the question: understanding time lags in translational research. J R Soc Med 2011;104(12):510–20.
29. Institute of Medicine. Crossing the quality chasm : a new health system for the 21st century. Washington, D.C.: National Academy Press; 2001.
30. Niven DJ, Rubenfeld GD, Kramer AA, et al. Effect of published scientific evidence on glycemic control in adult intensive care units. JAMA Intern Med 2015;175(5):801–9.

31. van der Vleuten CP, Schuwirth LW, Driessen EW, et al. A model for programmatic assessment fit for purpose. Med Teach 2012;34(3):205–14.
32. ten Cate O, Scheele F. Competency-based postgraduate training: can we bridge the gap between theory and clinical practice? Acad Med 2007;82(6): 542–7.
33. Malone K, Supri S. A critical time for medical education: the perils of competence-based reform of the curriculum. Adv Health Sci Educ Theory Pract 2012;17(2):241–6.
34. Halman S, Dudek N, Wood T, et al. Direct observation of clinical skills feedback scale: development and validity evidence. Teach Learn Med 2016;28(4): 385–94.
35. Miller A, Archer J. Impact of workplace based assessment on doctors' education and performance: a systematic review. BMJ 2010;341:c5064.
36. Schuwirth LW, Van der Vleuten CP. Programmatic assessment: from assessment of learning to assessment for learning. Med Teach 2011;33(6):478–85.
37. Al-Eraky M, Marei H. A fresh look at Miller's pyramid: assessment at the 'Is' and 'Do' levels. Med Educ 2016;50(12):1253–7.
38. Norcini J, Anderson MB, Bollela V, et al. 2018 Consensus framework for good assessment. Med Teach 2018;40(11):1–8.
39. Crossley J, Johnson G, Booth J, et al. Good questions, good answers: construct alignment improves the performance of workplace-based assessment scales. Med Educ 2011;45(6):560–9.
40. Ginsburg S, van der Vleuten CPM, Eva KW. The hidden value of narrative comments for assessment: a quantitative reliability analysis of qualitative data. Acad Med 2017;92(11):1617–21.
41. Ginsburg S, Regehr G, Lingard L, et al. Reading between the lines: faculty interpretations of narrative evaluation comments. Med Educ 2015;49(3):296–306.
42. Ginsburg S, Eva K, Regehr G. Do in-training evaluation reports deserve their bad reputations? A study of the reliability and predictive ability of ITER scores and narrative comments. Acad Med 2013;88(10):1539–44.
43. Ginsburg S, van der Vleuten CP, Eva KW, et al. Cracking the code: residents' interpretations of written assessment comments. Med Educ 2017;51(4):401–10.
44. Dudek NL, Marks MB, Wood TJ, et al. Assessing the quality of supervisors' completed clinical evaluation reports. Med Educ 2008;42(8):816–22.
45. Holmboe ES. Work-based assessment and co-production in postgraduate medical training. GMS J Med Educ 2017;34(5):Doc58.
46. Ten Cate TJ, Kusurkar RA, Williams GC. How self-determination theory can assist our understanding of the teaching and learning processes in medical education. AMEE guide No. 59. Med Teach 2011;33(12):961–73.
47. Sandars J, Cleary TJ. Self-regulation theory: applications to medical education: AMEE Guide No. 58. Med Teach 2011;33(11):875–86.
48. Young JQ, Sugarman R, Schwartz J, et al. A mobile app to capture EPA assessment data: utilizing the consolidated framework for implementation research to identify enablers and barriers to engagement. Perspect Med Educ 2020;9(4): 210–9.
49. Young JQ, Sugarman R, Schwartz J, et al. Faculty and resident engagement with a workplace-based assessment tool: use of implementation science to explore enablers and barriers. Acad Med 2020;95(12):1937–44.
50. Sargeant J, Mann K, van der Vleuten C, et al. "Directed" self-assessment: practice and feedback within a social context. J Contin Educ Health Prof 2008;28(1): 47–54.

51. Konings KD, van Berlo J, Koopmans R, et al. Using a smartphone app and coaching group sessions to promote residents' reflection in the workplace. Acad Med 2016;91(3):365–70.

52. LaDonna KA, Ginsburg S, Watling C. Rising to the level of your incompetence": what physicians' self-assessment of their performance reveals about the imposter syndrome in medicine. Acad Med 2018;93(5):763–8.

53. Schuwirth LW, van der Vleuten CP. Programmatic assessment and Kane's validity perspective. Med Educ 2012;46(1):38–48.

54. Van Der Vleuten CPM, Schuwirth LWT, Driessen EW, et al. Twelve Tips for programmatic assessment. Med Teach 2015;37(7):641–6.

55. Young JQ, Frank JR, Holmboe ES, et al. Advancing Workplace-Based Assessment in Psychiatric Education: Key Design and Implementation Issues. Psychiatry Clin 2021;44(2):317–32.

56. Padilla A, Benjamin S, Lewis-Fernandez R. Assessing cultural psychiatry milestones through an objective structured clinical examination. Acad Psychiatry 2016;40(4):600–3.

57. Young JQ, Lieu S, O'Sullivan P, et al. Development and initial testing of a structured clinical observation tool to assess pharmacotherapy competence. Acad Psychiatry 2011;35(1):27–34.

58. Young JQ, Irby DM, Kusz M, et al. Performance assessment of pharmacotherapy: results from a content validity survey of the psychopharmacotherapy-structured clinical observation (P-SCO) tool. Acad Psychiatry 2018;42(6): 765–72.

59. Young JQ, Rasul R, O'Sullivan PS. Evidence for the validity of the psychopharmacotherapy-structured clinical observation tool: results of a factor and time series analysis. Acad Psychiatry 2018;42(6):759–64.

60. Young JQ, Sugarman R, Holmboe E, et al. Advancing our understanding of narrative comments generated by direct observation tools: lessons from the psychopharmacotherapy-structured clinical observation. J Grad Med Educ 2019;11(5):570–9.

61. Jibson MD, Broquet KE, Anzia JM, et al. Clinical skills verification in general psychiatry: recommendations of the ABPN task force on rater training. Acad Psychiatry 2012;36(5):363–8.

62. Weiss A, Ozdoba A, Carroll V, et al. Entrustable professional activities: enhancing meaningful use of evaluations and milestones in a psychiatry residency program. Acad Psychiatry 2016;40(5):850–4.

63. Pinilla S, Lenouvel E, Strik W, et al. Entrustable professional activities in psychiatry: a systematic review. Acad Psychiatry 2020;44(1):37–45.

64. Kogan JR, Conforti LN, Bernabeo E, et al. How faculty members experience workplace-based assessment rater training: a qualitative study. Med Educ 2015;49(7):692–708.

65. van de Ridder JM, McGaghie WC, Stokking KM, et al. Variables that affect the process and outcome of feedback, relevant for medical training: a meta-review. Med Educ 2015;49(7):658–73.

66. Sargeant J, Lockyer JM, Mann K, et al. The R2C2 model in residency education: how does it foster coaching and promote feedback use? Acad Med 2018;93(7): 1055–63.

67. Holmboe EH. Developing faculty competencies in assessment. Available at: https://www.acgme.org/Meetings-and-Educational-Activities/Other-Educational-Activities/Courses-and-Workshops/Developing-Faculty-Competencies-in-Assessment. Accessed May 20, 2020.

68. Iobst WI, Holmboe ES. Programmatic assessment: the secret sauce of effective CBME implementation. J Grad Med Educ 2020;12(4):518–21.
69. Eva KW. On the generality of specificity. Med Educ 2003;37(7):587–8.
70. van der Vleuten CP, Schuwirth LW. Assessing professional competence: from methods to programmes. Med Educ 2005;39(3):309–17.
71. Eva KW, Bordage G, Campbell C, et al. Towards a program of assessment for health professionals: from training into practice. Adv Health Sci Educ Theory Pract 2016;21(4):897–913.
72. Thoma B, Bandi V, Carey R, et al. Developing a dashboard to meet competence committee needs: a design-based research project. Can Med Educ J 2020; 11(1):e16–34.
73. Warm EJ, Kinnear B, Kelleher M, et al. Transforming resident assessment: an analysis using Deming's system of profound knowledge. Acad Med 2018; 94(2):195–201.
74. Warm EJ, Held JD, Hellmann M, et al. Entrusting observable practice activities and milestones over the 36 months of an internal medicine residency. Acad Med 2016;91(10):1398–405.
75. Ross S, Binczyk NM, Hamza DM, et al. Association of a competency-based assessment system with identification of and support for medical residents in difficulty. JAMA Netw Open 2018;1(7):e184581.
76. Holmboe ES, Yamazaki K, Nasca TJ, et al. Using longitudinal milestones data and learning analytics to facilitate the professional development of residents: early lessons from three specialties. Acad Med 2020;95(1):97–103.
77. Warm EJ. Personal Communication. January 27, 2020.
78. Govaerts M. Workplace-based assessment and assessment for learning: threats to validity. J Grad Med Educ 2015;7(2):265–7.
79. Watling CJ, Kenyon CF, Zibrowski EM, et al. Rules of engagement: residents' perceptions of the in-training evaluation process. Acad Med 2008;83(10 Suppl):S97–100.
80. Nicol DJ, Macfarlane-Dick D. Formative assessment and self-regulated learning: a model and seven principles of good feedback practice. Studies in Higher Education 2006;31(2):199–218.
81. Watling C, LaDonna KA, Lingard L, et al. Sometimes the work just needs to be done': socio-cultural influences on direct observation in medical training. Med Educ 2016;50(10):1054–64.
82. Harrison CJ, Konings KD, Molyneux A, et al. Web-based feedback after summative assessment: how do students engage? Med Educ 2013;47(7):734–44.
83. Young JQ, Sugarman R, Schwartz J, et al. Using implementation science to explore the enablers and barriers to engagement with a direct observation and feedback tool. Acad Med 2020;95(12):1937–44.
84. White CB, Gruppen LD, Fantone JC. Self-regulated learning in medical education. In: Understanding Medical Education. 2013:201–11.
85. Sargeant J, Lockyer J, Mann K, et al. Facilitated reflective performance feedback: developing an evidence- and theory-based model that builds relationship, explores reactions and content, and coaches for performance change (R2C2). Acad Med 2015;90(12):1698–706.
86. Gawande A. Personal best: top athletes and singers have coaches. Should you? New Yorker. 2011. Available at: http://www.newyorker.com/magazine/2011/10/03/personal-best. Accessed April 1, 2020.

87. Ericsson KA. Acquisition and maintenance of medical expertise: a perspective from the expert-performance approach with deliberate practice. Acad Med 2015;90(11):1471–86.

88. Palamara K, Kauffman C, Stone VE, et al. Promoting success: a professional development coaching program for interns in medicine. J Grad Med Educ 2015;7(4):630–7.

89. Parks K, Miller J, Westcott A. Coaching in graduate medical education. In: coaching in medical education: a faculty handbook. American Medical Association 2017;50–3.

90. Telio S, Regehr G, Ajjawi R. Feedback and the educational alliance: examining credibility judgements and their consequences. Med Educ 2016;50(9):933–42.

91. Sargeant J, Eva KW, Armson H, et al. Features of assessment learners use to make informed self-assessments of clinical performance. Med Educ 2011; 45(6):636–47.

92. Hauer KE, Chesluk B, Iobst W, et al. Reviewing residents' competence: a qualitative study of the role of clinical competency committees in performance assessment. Acad Med 2015;90(8):1084–92.

93. Andolesk K, Padmore J, Hauer KE, et al. Clinical competency committees: a guidebook for programs. Accreditation council for graduate medical education. 2020. Available at: file:///C:/Users/jyoung9/OneDrive%20-%20Northwell%20Health/Academic/Presentations%20and%20Publications/Psychiatric%20Clinics/System%20Article/ACGMEClinicalCompetencyCommitteeGuidebook%20(1).pdf. Accessed May 20, 2020.

94. Teherani A, Hauer KE, Fernandez A, et al. How small differences in assessed clinical performance amplify to large differences in grades and awards: a cascade with serious consequences for students underrepresented in medicine. Acad Med 2018;93(9):1286–92.

95. Klein R, Julian KA, Snyder ED, et al. Gender bias in resident assessment in graduate medical education: review of the literature. J Gen Intern Med 2019; 34(5):712–9.

96. Rojek AE, Khanna R, Yim JWL, et al. Differences in narrative language in evaluations of medical students by gender and under-represented minority status. J Gen Intern Med 2019;34(5):684–91.

97. Donato AA, Alweis R, Wenderoth S. Design of a clinical competency committee to maximize formative feedback. J Community Hosp Intern Med Perspect 2016; 6(6):33533.

98. Schwind CJ, Williams RG, Boehler ML, et al. Do individual attendings' post-rotation performance ratings detect residents' clinical performance deficiencies? Acad Med 2004;79(5):453–7.

99. Pack R, Lingard L, Watling CJ, et al. Some assembly required: tracing the interpretative work of Clinical Competency Committees. Med Educ 2019;53(7): 723–34.

100. Hauer KE, Cate OT, Boscardin CK, et al. Ensuring resident competence: a narrative review of the literature on group decision making to inform the work of clinical competency committees. J Grad Med Educ 2016;8(2):156–64.

101. Kinnear B, Warm EJ, Hauer KE. Twelve tips to maximize the value of a clinical competency committee in postgraduate medical education. Med Teach 2018; 40(11):1110–5.

102. Birken SA, Powell BJ, Presseau J, et al. Combined use of the consolidated framework for implementation research (CFIR) and the theoretical domains framework (TDF): a systematic review. Implement Sci 2017;12(1):2.
103. Bowe CM, Armstrong E. Assessment for systems learning: a holistic assessment framework to support decision making across the medical education continuum. Acad Med 2017;92(5):585–92.
104. Warm EJ, Edgar L, Kelleher M, et al. A guidebook for implementing and changing assessment in the milestone era. Accreditation council for graduate medical education. 2020. Available at: https://www.acgme.org/Portals/0/Milestones%20Implementation%202020.pdf?ver=2020-05-11-165927-097. Accessed May 1, 2020.

Giving Feedback

Hermioni L. Amonoo, MD, MPP[a,b,c,]*, Regina M. Longley, BA[d],
Diana M. Robinson, MD[e,f]

KEYWORDS

- Feedback • Medical education • Clinical competence • Evaluation
- Psychiatric education • Educational milestones

KEY POINTS

- Effective feedback is fundamental to psychiatric training, as it promotes progression through educational milestones, informs students about learning style preferences, and sparks improved clinical competence.
- It is essential to consider feedback-giver characteristics that are heavily valued by the feedback receiver, who ultimately determines how the feedback is perceived and used.
- We must recognize barriers to constructive receipt of feedback, including truth, relationship, and identity triggers, which can precipitate unproductive emotional reactions, feelings of insecurity, and sense of threat to identity on the part of the feedback receiver.
- Feedback givers and receivers should adopt a "growth identity," understanding that we are a work-in-progress and focusing on nurturing our shortcomings to generate advancement.

INTRODUCTION

Effective feedback is essential to medical education for myriad reasons. Feedback promotes learning and ensures that benchmarks for various learning objectives are achieved.[1] Feedback also provides opportunities for learners to gain insights about their learning style, strengths, weaknesses, and progress on educational milestones. Effective feedback highlights dissonance between the intended result and the actual outcome and provides growth opportunities for learners to reflect on their learning process. Effective feedback presents information rather than judgements about observations, concerns, and behaviors with the sole purpose of the recipient improving performance.

[a] Department of Psychiatry, Brigham and Women's Hospital, 60 Fenwood Road, 4th Floor, Boston, MA 02115, USA; [b] Department of Psychosocial Oncology and Palliative Care, Dana-Farber Cancer Institute, Boston, MA, USA; [c] Harvard Medical School, Boston, MA, USA; [d] Department of Psychiatry, Massachusetts General Hospital, 125 Nashua Street, Suite #324, Boston, MA 02114, USA; [e] Department of Psychiatry, Parkland Hospital, Dallas, TX, USA; [f] UT Southwestern Medical School, 5323 Harry Hines Boulevard, Dallas, TX 75390, USA
* Corresponding author. Department of Psychiatry, Brigham and Women's Hospital, 60 Fenwood Road, 4th Floor, Boston, MA 02115.
E-mail address: hermioni_amonoo@dfci.harvard.edu

Psychiatr Clin N Am 44 (2021) 237–247
https://doi.org/10.1016/j.psc.2020.12.006
0193-953X/21/© 2020 Elsevier Inc. All rights reserved.

Extensive research over the past decade has proposed many definitions for effective feedback.[2] Effective feedback always provides an impetus for change or reinforces good clinical practice.[3] Effective feedback should always provide the trainee with tools to improve performance or bolster behaviors that contribute to clinical competence. Ultimately, effective feedback is a virtuous cycle of giving, where a teacher or supervisor provides learners the essential gift of insight into how to further advance their skills. Lack of feedback in a learning cycle results in stunted growth that can have downstream negative implications on clinical care. Although most feedback is understood in the context of learners receiving feedback from faculty and supervisors, anecdotal evidence supports that feedback provided by learners to their faculty can also be an underestimated source of faculty development.

The nature and response to feedback is varied. Feedback can be negative, positive, neutral, constructive or destructive, and in-depth or insignificant depending on multiple factors including prior experience with receiving or giving feedback. Positive responses to feedback stem from prior useful learning or formative experience from constructive feedback, whereas negative reactions are likely due to an association with a bad or judgmental experience with the feedback process. Despite varying responses to feedback, it can still provide an opportunity for people to correct misconceptions and reinforce good clinical practice that promotes competence.

In psychiatric education, effective feedback is especially critical considering the subjective nature of various aspects of the specialty. Critiques can easily be considered judgmental as compared with other procedural fields in medicine where specific skills have more objective benchmarks. Unfortunately, the nature of psychiatric practice presents challenges to providing effective feedback and evidence supports that psychiatric learners express not receiving sufficient feedback to promote their growth and development in psychiatric training.[4] The authors' observations in psychiatry regrettably resonate with Jack Ende's observations in 1983 that feedback is often omitted and handled inappropriately in clinical settings despite how essential it is.[3] Ende goes on to provide guidelines on how to give feedback, borrowing principles from business administration, psychology, and education.[3] Accordingly, in this article, the authors provide a comprehensive review and overview of effective feedback and offer suggestions for how it can be implemented and used in psychiatric education.

THE EFFECTIVE FEEDBACK PROCESS

The effective feedback process entails a supportive conversation that clarifies awareness of one's developing competencies, enhances self-efficacy and self-awareness for making progress, reinforces good clinical practices, identifies omissions, challenges a set of objectives for improvement, and facilitates development of strategies to enable that improvement to occur. Effective feedback occurs as part of a social interaction influenced by culture, values, expectations, personal histories, relationships, and power. Feedback, therefore, is not a one-way conversation but rather a discussion between the 2 parties involved. The feedback conversation is more effective with planning: (1) givers of feedback plan on the critical take-away points to be conveyed in the conversation; (2) receivers plan on the kinds of feedback and topics they want to add to the conversation's agenda.

There are many classifications of feedback. Branch, Paranjape, Hesketh, and Laidlaw articulate that feedback can be brief/informal or extensive/formal. Brief feedback is 5 minutes or less, whereas extensive feedback is 15 minutes or longer. Brief feedback is more about every day clinical interactions given in the context of work. It is frequent and given in small quantities/nuggets (ie, 1 to 2 high-yield takeaways), which allows problems to be detected early. Extensive feedback, on the other hand, can be over a period of time or after an entire learning experience.[5,6] Further, effective feedback can be approached in several ways including the sandwich model, the ask-tell-ask model, and reflective feedback conversation. **Table 1** summarizes common feedback approaches used in medical education as well as some pros and cons of each approach.

Anyone who makes a valid observation of a trainee's performance and has gathered enough data from his or her experience with the trainee can provide feedback, making the source of feedback givers wide-ranging, including peers, supervisors, patients, and other clinicians. Irrespective of the person, the source providing the feedback has to be credible and well intentioned, as this can affect how the feedback is provided and how the recipient is affected. Although patients cannot provide technical feedback, they can give important feedback on the relationship between patient and doctor and also provide insights on perceived empathy from their interaction with the clinical team.

Culture affects how learners perceive the instructiveness of feedback. Suhoyo and colleagues[12,13] explored the differences in the feedback process and perceived instructiveness among 215 Indonesian students. They found that students perceived feedback to be more instructive if it came from their attending physician equivalent compared with other sources. Conversely, a similar study by Van Hell and colleagues[14] in the Netherlands showed that Dutch students appreciated feedback more if it was based on observation regardless of the source. Further, feedback on directly observed behavior was perceived to be more instructive than feedback on information not observed.[14] Hence, effective feedback should reflect some of these factors; it should contain concrete and specific information, have irrefutable data and observations, focus on behaviors and actions rather than the learner, be limited to remediable behavior, and contain suggestions for improvement. An example of specific feedback is as follows: "I had a great deal of trouble following your biopsychosocial formulation today" versus "You were very disorganized in your presentation of the formulation." Although the first statement focuses on an observation, the second statement can easily be interpreted as an attack on the learner.

When feedback is given can be important. Effective feedback should ideally not be given randomly rather when learners are prepared. The closer it is in proximity to the performance or observation, the more effective it is. Also, effective feedback should be given in a psychologically safe environment, whether in private or public, and the context should be carefully examined. Feedback presented as a discussion allows for interaction and response. Effective feedback blends positive and negative information in a thoughtful way, and, overall, both parties should work together as allies for the common goal of helping the learner improve. Contrary to popular belief that face-to-face feedback is more effective, in a single blind, randomized controlled trial at 2 university-based internal medicine residency programs, Elnicki and colleagues[15] found there were no significant differences in oral versus written feedback, indicating aspects other than delivery of the feedback should be assessed.

BARRIERS TO EFFECTIVE FEEDBACK

Now that we have defined what feedback is, who is involved, what it contains, when it is best discussed, and how to best discuss it, we build on this to look at common barriers to effective feedback. Feedback can be further broken down into appreciation, coaching, and evaluation. We need all 3 types of feedback to satisfy different learning needs. Appreciation is recognition from the feedback receivers to the feedback givers

Table 1
Examples of approaches to feedback

Approach	Description	Pros	Cons
Sandwich model[7,8]	This technique delivers negative criticisms sandwiched between positive comments	• Reinforces positive feedback • Can be brief • Applicable in most clinical encounters	• Feedback receiver is passive • Does not always consider the relationships between the individuals • Usually reports on single events • When used continuously, can lose its effectiveness • Feedback receivers may overly fixate on negative or positive comments
Pendleton model[9]	This technique entails asking trainees to reflect and highlight on positive and negative clinical behaviors, whereas feedback giver reinforces positive behaviors and provides suggestions for how to improve weaknesses or modify certain behaviors	• Actively engages the learner • Learner sets agenda and feedback giver builds on it • Covers both positive and negative comments • Identifies action plans and goals	• Because learner sets the agenda, may not be as comprehensive • Requires that the learner has good insight about their performance
Ask-tell-ask model[10]	This technique encourages trainee's reflection and self-assessment of their skills in 3 steps: • Ask—for trainee's self-assessment; • Tell—entails providing observations, focused teaching, and feedback on what trainee has stated and; • Ask—for trainee's understanding and develop a plan of action	• Learner-centered, specific feedback • Dialogue where both giver and receiver contribute to the agenda • Develops a plan for improvement	• Requires preparation and time for both parties • Requires trainees have insights about their skills to inform the conversation • Time intensive if 3 steps are actively pursued

(continued on next page)

Table 1
(continued)

Approach	Description	Pros	Cons
Feedforward model	This technique is future oriented and provides learners with suggestions and tips on what the learning experience entails to foster reinforceable behaviors	• Potentially minimizes learners' engagement in undesirable behaviors • Forward oriented, unlike most feedback that relies on previous information • Less likely to be judgmental, as learners are yet to experience learning environment	• Learners are passive • Requires faculty to have significant familiarity with learning environment to provide practical suggestions for learners
R2C2[11]	This technique is structured around: • Relationship—relationship and rapport building; • Reaction—exploring previous reactions to feedback; • Content—exploring feedback content; • Coaching—coaching for change	• Focuses on rapport building and 2-way feedback conversation • Learners are actively and reflectively engaged • Provides specific phrasing to help facilitate each phase • Coaching aspect was found to be helpful to residents and supervisors[11]	• Time intensive (feedback sessions lasted 20 min) • Proof-of-concept study was done with residents who were all performing well, so more studies will need to look at the effectiveness of this approach with struggling residents

that they and their efforts are seen, heard, and understood. It is critical to building human relationships, rapport, and motivation. Coaching is advising on how a certain procedure/task/interaction can be done better or in a different way, whereas evaluation is discussion of where someone stands in relation to peers or specific metrics (such as the Graduate Medical Education milestones). Coaching is ideally based on recent, specific, observed, constructive, actionable information and is given in the context of a trusting relationship, whereas evaluations are more summative. However, with the complexities of the training environment where trainees may work with multiple attending physicians for varying lengths of time, the actual circumstances can fall short of the ideal for feedback provision.

Before effective feedback of any type can be given, it is helpful for the feedback giver and receiver to be specific about what feedback they are giving and hoping to receive. When there is a mismatch between these 2, it is helpful to take a step back to clarify which type of feedback this is. When possible, it is ideal to stick to giving one kind of feedback, but occasionally coaching and evaluation are delivered at the same time. When this happens, the evaluation portion can drown out the coaching portion. It is important not to assume what a trainee wants to learn, why a trainee is struggling, if a trainee wants feedback, what information the trainee will take out of a feedback conversation, or if they intend to incorporate the feedback. Thus, asking questions, making a plan for when to follow-up on the feedback and anticipating possible consequences that may occur from not taking the feedback (ie, clarifying when performance is suboptimal vs a different way of approaching the problem) are essential.[16] Additional barriers to feedback are due to factors specific to the feedback giver, receiver, or both (**Table 2**).

FACTORS RELATED TO THE FEEDBACK GIVER

In a survey study of the feedback factors most valued by US psychiatry residents, most of the residents strongly valued evaluators who modeled feedback giving skills.[17] Other feedback giver skills that were shown to influence receptivity included role modeling, clinical skills, and interpersonal skills.[16–19] Of note, trainees may apply indirect proxies for engagement in the feedback process such as if feedback evaluations are completed in a timely manner.[19,20] The specific timing may vary on the competence level of the trainee and the complexity of the task, and this most

Table 2 Different types of feedback			
	Appreciation	**Coaching**	**Evaluation**
Definition	To see, acknowledge, connect, motivate, thank.	To give receiver information, sharpen skills, and improve capability, not to judge.	To judge, assess, rate, or rank against a set of standards.
Endpoint	Satisfies the need to build relationships.	Satisfies the need to guide learning.	Satisfies the need to know where we stand, to set expectations, to feel reassured and secure, and to inform decision-making.
Assessment		Formative	Summative
Goal Orientation		Allows trainee to remain on course to reaching a goal	Provides information on how well a trainee reaches a goal in comparison to the performance of other peers
Statement type		Expressed as neutral statements	Expressed as normative statements
Grammatical structure		Composed of nouns and verbs	Composed of adjectives and adverbs
Time-frame		Continuous process of performance monitoring	Episodic and usually midpoint or end of an activity
Specificity		Regulated to quantities that are remediable	Comprehensive and detailed

frequently occurs soon after a patient encounter. Giving the feedback during the task can be seen as belittling or erodes the patient's confidence in the trainee or the trainee's confidence in themselves.[16,19,20] Multiple studies reiterated the importance of the feedback giver being approachable, supportive, and trustworthy to improve how feedback is received.[17–19,21] Feedback givers can nurture this relationship with setting and communicating clear expectations and making feedback an expected part of feedback receivers' rotations.[16,18,21] Feedback receivers also strongly value specific feedback based off the trainee's directly observed work.[16–20] With no evidence on the superiority of one feedback approach over another, it is preferable to use a personalized approach to the feedback giver and receiver and the situation.[16]

FACTORS RELATED TO THE FEEDBACK RECEIVER

Although the current feedback and learning literature has traditionally focused on improving the quality and abilities of the feedback giver, over the last 30 years there has been an increased focus on the feedback receiver. Ultimately, the feedback receiver is the gatekeeper for how the feedback is perceived and how they will use (or not use) it. In the seminal text on improving feedback receiving skills "Thanks for the Feedback," Stone and Heen identified 3 common areas of feedback barriers including truth triggers, relationship triggers, and identity triggers.[22]

First, truth triggers describe our emotional reactions to feedback that seems incorrect or unhelpful. Ways to overcome truth triggers include separating and identifying what type of feedback is happening (appreciation, coaching, or evaluation), understanding the feedback fully (moving past vague labels to understand where both groups are coming from), and coming from a place of curiosity to learn more instead of seeking to deflect the feedback by looking for what's wrong with it.[18,22] Everyone has blind spots where other people may hold the keys to seeing the whole picture more clearly.[22] Even when feedback is delivered suboptimally and in a less than ideal situation, an astute feedback receiver can find the kernel of truth that sparks valuable learning.[18]

Second, relationship triggers can come up due to the credibility/trust barrier in the dyadic relationship between giver and receiver or the feedback bringing up unresolved issues about appreciation among other relationship dynamics.[22] Solutions to work through these barriers include watching out for "switchtracking," when one topic (eg, "Here's how you can do this better this time") can quickly diverge into 2 topics (eg, "You don't appreciate how hard I've worked on this rotation). One must first listen, to identify that this has happened, then work together with the other party involved to set and prioritize the agenda to give adequate time to address and disentangle both topics.[22] Also, to see relationship triggers in action, both parties should take a step back to perceive what they are contributing to the situations that are prompting the feedback exchange.

Third, identity triggers explain how the feedback can feel threatening to an individual's identity with varying reactions, temperaments, and cognitive distortions.[22] Identity triggers include the accuracy of the information, how helpful the information is, and how pertinent the information is to the receiver. Solutions to identify triggers require feedback givers and receivers to reflect on how they respond to positive and negative feedback and recognize baseline temperaments that play a role in our sense of self. Shifting to a cognitive behavioral therapy mindset to recognize cognitive distortions at play can help transition an emotionally escalating situation back to a manageable size. Common cognitive distortions include all-or-nothing thinking, overgeneralization, focusing on a single negative piece of information to the exclusion of other information, disqualifying positive information, jumping to conclusions (mind reading—the inaccurate belief of knowing what the other person is thinking; and fortune telling—to draw conclusions and predictions from little or no information), catastrophizing/minimizing, emotional reading ("I feel it, therefore it must be true"), should statements, labeling, and personalization.[23]

In order to expand our ability to grow, feedback givers and receivers should cultivate a "growth identity," in which we are depicted as works in progress and seek to improve on wherever we are currently, as opposed to a "fixed identity" in which we are understood as the final (and best) version of ourselves. Immersed in a "fixed identity," feedback is received as unnecessary and confrontational to our current self. In a survey study of 166 obstetrics and gynecology residents and medical students,

---

Box 1
Toolkit for improving feedback skills

Improving Feedback Giving and Communication Skills
- Fisher R, Ury W, & Patton B. Getting to Yes: Negotiating Agreement Without Giving In (3rd ed.). New York, NY: Penguin Books; 2011.[25]
  - Short and clear resource on basic concepts of principled negation; particularly helpful with identifying underlying interests that inform positions and creative problem solving to generate multiple ways to satisfy both people's interests.
- Stone D, Patton B, & Heen S. Difficult conversations: How to discuss what matters most. New York, NY: Penguin Books; 2000.[26]
  - Guiding conversations to create mutual understanding of an issue so that you can both figure out the best way forward.
- Ury W. Getting Past No: Negotiating with Difficult People. New York: Bantam Books; 1991.[27]
  - Helpful strategies for negotiating with uncooperative people that are applicable to improving communication skills.
- Fisher R, Shapiro D. Beyond Reason: Using Emotions as You Negotiate. New York, NY: Viking Penguin; 2005.[28]
  - Helpful strategies for understanding negative emotions and engendering positive emotions in formal and informal negotiations that are applicable to improving communication skills.

Improving Feedback Receiving Skills
- Stone D, Heen S. Thanks for the feedback: The science and art of receiving feedback well (even when it is off base, unfair, poorly delivered, and, frankly, you're not in the mood). UK: Portfolio Penguin; 2015.[22]
  - High-yield resource on navigating common barriers that make it difficult to receive and implement feedback, especially how to nurture a personal growth identity.
  - Authors' online team leader discussion guide is helpful for facilitating journal clubs, book clubs, and team building.
- https://stoneandheen.com/sites/stoneandheen.com/files/TFTF%20Team%20Leaders%20bv2-1b.pdf
- Ury W. The Power of a Positive No: Save the Deal, Save the Relationship, and Still Say No. New York, NY: Bantam Books; 2008.[29]
  - Provides specific strategies and examples for learning to say "no" that are applicable to many situations.
- Beck JS. Cognitive behavior therapy: Basics and beyond (2nd ed.). Guilford Press; 2011.[23]
  - Particularly helpful for identifying cognitive distortions and how to manage them.

Improving Institutional Cultures of Feedback
- Batista E. Building a Feedback-Rich Culture. Harvard Business Review. 2013 Dec 24 [cited 2020 May 20]; Available from: https://hbr.org/2013/12/building-a-feedback-rich-culture.[30]
- Ernst R. Council Post: Three Steps For Creating A Feedback Culture. Forbes. [cited 2020 May 20]. Available from: https://www.forbes.com/sites/forbeshumanresourcescouncil/2019/01/03/three-steps-for-creating-a-feedback-culture/.[31]

residents with a higher learning goal orientation were more likely to ask for feedback and perceived greater benefits with fewer costs. Conversely, residents with a fixed mindset were less likely to ask for feedback and more likely to read into indirect signs that support their performance.[21] A "growth identity" is comparable to having a mindset that seeks out and incorporates coaching, commonly adopted by top athletes, singers, and outlined by surgeon Dr Atul Gawande in *Better*.[18,22,24] It is also important to consider that the feedback dyad occurs in the context of a larger culture of learning (or lack thereof), which affects how willing both parties are to take the time, energy, and concern to anticipate how the feedback may be taken (**Box 1**). The next section will explore the culture of learning in greater detail.

CREATING A CULTURE OF FEEDBACK/CLINICAL CARE POINTS

There is increased evidence examining how institutions can create a culture of feedback and learning. The following are evidence-based pearls and pitfalls for feedback givers relevant to nurturing a culture of feedback.

- Model the types of behavior they are wanting to instill (especially from the top).[16,17,22]
  - Example: trainees should be encouraged to give feedback to their supervisors, and their supervisors should model how to receive and process it.
- Make role modeling deliberate, explicit, and frequent.
- Build feedback into a systems-based approach throughout the learning process.[16,20]
- Make sure that teams give feedback regularly and follow refresher courses to maintain and improve competency in providing feedback.[16]
- Do not rely exclusively on faculty development to improve effectiveness of feedback.[16]
- Nurture relationship between faculty and trainees to establish a foundation of trust, support, and approachability.
- Personalize feedback to trainee's goals to improve motivation.
- Give collaborative feedback (have the receiver reflect on their performance during the feedback encounter).
- Think beyond the feedback sandwich—there are lots of other approaches to giving feedback, and a more flexible approach is helpful.

SUMMARY

Effective feedback is a fundamental aspect of psychiatric training, as it promotes progression through educational milestones, informs students about preferences in learning styles, and sparks improvement in clinical competence. There are many approaches to providing feedback, all of which target and prove advantageous for different aspects of the feedback dynamic such as learner engagement and minimization of judgment. It is also essential to consider the implications of characteristics related to the feedback giver (eg, role modeling, feedback skills, and clinical skills) that are heavily valued by the feedback receiver, who is ultimately the determining factor in how the feedback is perceived and used. The feedback receiver role, though, is not passive, and it is imperative that we recognize potential barriers to constructive receipt of the feedback, including truth, relationship, and identity triggers, which can precipitate unproductive emotional reactions, feelings of insecurity, and sense of threat to identity on the part of the feedback receiver. In order to combat these barriers, feedback givers and receivers alike should adopt a "growth identity," understanding that we are a work-in-progress and focusing on nurturing our short-comings to generate advancement. Ultimately, a concerted effort by feedback givers and receivers founded on a sense of trust, support, and approachability is vital for establishing a culture of feedback in psychiatric education.

DISCLOSURE

The authors have nothing to disclose.

REFERENCES

1. Hewson MG, Little ML. Giving feedback in medical education: verification of recommended techniques. J Gen Intern Med 1998;13(2):111–6.
2. Bing-You R, Hayes V, Varaklis K, et al. Feedback for learners in medical education: what is known? A scoping review. Acad Med 2017;92(9):1346–54.
3. Ende J. Feedback in clinical medical education. JAMA 1983;250(6):777–81.
4. Brown N, Cooke L. Giving effective feedback to psychiatric trainees. Adv Psychiatr Treat 2009;15:123–8.
5. Branch WT Jr, Paranjape A. Feedback and reflection: teaching methods for clinical settings. Acad Med 2002;77(12 Pt 1):1185–8.
6. Hesketh EA, Laidlaw JM. Developing the teaching instinct, 1: feedback. Med Teach 2002;24(3):245–8.
7. Brown LE, Rangachari D, Melia M. Beyond the sandwich: from feedback to clinical coaching for residents as teachers. MedEdPORTAL 2017;13:10627.
8. Dohrenwend A. Serving up the feedback sandwich. Fam Pract Manag 2002; 9(10):43–6.
9. Hardavella G, Aamli-Gaagnat A, Saad N, et al. How to give and receive feedback effectively. Breathe (Sheff) 2017;13(4):327–33.
10. French JC, Colbert CY, Pien LC, et al. Targeted feedback in the milestones era: utilization of the ask-tell-ask feedback model to promote reflection and self-assessment. J Surg Educ 2015;72(6):e274–9.
11. Sargeant J, Mann K, Manos S, et al. R2C2 in action: testing an evidence-based model to facilitate feedback and coaching in residency. J Grad Med Educ 2017; 9(2):165–70.
12. Suhoyo Y, Schonrock-Adema J, Emilia O, et al. Clinical workplace learning: perceived learning value of individual and group feedback in a collectivistic culture. BMC Med Educ 2018;18(1):79.
13. Suhoyo Y, van Hell EA, Prihatiningsih TS, et al. Exploring cultural differences in feedback processes and perceived instructiveness during clerkships: replicating a Dutch study in Indonesia. Med Teach 2014;36(3):223–9.
14. Van Hell EA, Kuks JB, Raat AN, et al. Instructiveness of feedback during clerkships: influence of supervisor, observation and student initiative. Med Teach 2009;31(1):45–50.
15. Elnicki DM, Layne RD, Ogden PE, et al. Oral versus written feedback in medical clinic. J Gen Intern Med 1998;13(3):155–8.
16. Lefroy J, Watling C, Teunissen PW, et al. Guidelines: the do's, don'ts and don't knows of feedback for clinical education. Perspect Med Educ 2015;4(6):284–99.
17. Beaulieu AM, Kim BS, Topor DR, et al. Seeing is believing: an exploration of what residents value when they receive feedback. Acad Psychiatry 2019;43(5): 507–11.

18. Reddy ST, Zegarek MH, Fromme HB, et al. Barriers and facilitators to effective feedback: a qualitative analysis of data from multispecialty resident focus groups. J Grad Med Educ 2015;7(2):214–9.
19. Watling CJ, Kenyon CF, Zibrowski EM, et al. Rules of engagement: residents' perceptions of the in-training evaluation process. Acad Med 2008;83(10 Suppl): S97–100.
20. Cantillon P, Sargeant J. Giving feedback in clinical settings. BMJ 2008;337: a1961.
21. Teunissen PW, Stapel DA, van der Vleuten C, et al. Who wants feedback? An investigation of the variables influencing residents' feedback-seeking behavior in relation to night shifts. Acad Med 2009;84(7):910–7.
22. Stone D, Heen S. Thanks for the feedback : the science and art of receiving feedback well : (even when it is off base, unfair, poorly delivered, and frankly, you're not in the mood). United Kingdom: Portfolio Penguin; 2015.
23. Beck JS. Cognitive behavior therapy : basics and beyond. New York (London): Guilford; 2011.
24. Gawande A. Better : a surgeon's notes on performance. New York (NY): Metropolitan; 2007.
25. Ury W, Patton B, Fisher R. Getting to yes : negotiating agreement without giving in. 3rd edition, revised edition. New York, N.Y.: Penguin Books; 2011.
26. Patton B, Heen S, Stone D. Difficult conversations : how to discuss what matters most. New York, N.Y.: Penguin Books; 2000.
27. Ury W. Getting past no : negotiating with difficult people. New York (NY): Bantam Books; 1991.
28. Shapiro D, Fisher R. Beyond reason : using emotions as you negotiate. New York (NY): Viking; 2005.
29. Ury W. The power of a positive no : how to say no and still get to yes ; [save the deal, save the relationship - and still say no]. New York (NY): Bantam Books; 2008.
30. Batista E. Building a feedback-rich culture. Harv Bus Rev 2013.
31. Ernst R. Three Steps for Creating A Feedback Culture. In. Forbes: Forbes Human Research Council; 2019.

Multiple-Choice Tests: A–Z in Best Writing Practices

Vikas Gupta, MD, MPH[a], Eric R. Williams, MD[b],*, Roopma Wadhwa, MD, MHA[a]

KEYWORDS

- Multiple-choice questions • MCQs • Assessment • Multiple-choice tests
- Standards • Guidelines • Psychiatry assessment

KEY POINTS

- Multiple-choice questions (MCQs) are popular as assessment tools in psychiatry and medical education.
- Guidelines based on best practice and evidence can help with creating high-quality MCQs.
- Vignettes are useful in assessing complex problem solving and higher-order thinking.
- Faculty must familiarize themselves with best practices in writing MCQs.
- High-quality MCQs enhance the validity and reliability of assessment examinations.

INTRODUCTION

Multiple-choice questions (MCQs) are a time-honored method for assessing test takers. These assessments can reveal areas of strengths and weaknesses in examinees and training programs and can provide useful feedback for improvement.[1] Appropriately designed multiple-choice questions result in an unbiased assessment that can test knowledge, comprehension, application, and analysis.[2]

Multiple-choice tests are stronger predictors of student performance than other types of evaluations, such as in-class participation, written assignments, case examinations, and simulation games.[3] MCQs are useful to assess for higher-order thinking, including application, analysis, evaluation, and creation of knowledge.[4] Testing agencies can administer them to thousands of examinees; they can test a vast body of knowledge and are easy to score. They are useful as a learning tool and effective for learning about tested information and competitive information related to incorrect alternatives.[5] However, few psychiatrists have training in writing high-quality MCQs. There is limited literature in psychiatry on writing MCQs, and this article is an update to an article previously published in 2010 by Boland and colleagues.[6]

[a] South Carolina Department of Mental Health, 2715 Colonial Drive, Suite 200-A, Colonial Drive, Columbia, SC 29201, USA; [b] University of South Carolina School of Medicine, 6311 Garners Ferry Road, Suite 126, Columbia, SC 29209, USA
* Corresponding author.
E-mail address: Eric.Williams@uscmed.sc.edu

Psychiatr Clin N Am 44 (2021) 249–261
https://doi.org/10.1016/j.psc.2021.03.008
0193-953X/21/© 2021 Elsevier Inc. All rights reserved.

HISTORY AND BACKGROUND

Medical examinations since the 1950s have been using MCQs.[7] Formal training for writing MCQs leads to writing questions with fewer flaws.[8] An evaluation of MCQs in a hospital learning management system revealed one deficit in half of the items, more than one fault in nearly a third, and only approximately 15% of the questions were flawless.[9] Other published articles have shown flaw rates as high as 80%.[10] Item-writing flaws lead to greater difficulty and lower discrimination[11] with no increase in item discrimination between higher-performing and lower-performing test-takers.[12] Also, faulty items may lead to increased failure rates due to the introduction of extraneous factors. Training for question writers leads to the increased cognitive level of the questions[13] progressing from measuring declarative knowledge to procedural knowledge, especially with the aid of an interdisciplinary review committee.

Different item-writing flaws are associated with varying effects on test-takers. Longer correct answers, implausible distractors, and eponymous terms positively impact scores, whereas having the central idea in the choices rather than the stem negatively impacts scores.[14] When items were analyzed for flaws and feedback given to item writers, the number of flaws decreased proportionately to the amount of time before the test was delivered.[15]

STANDARDS

Examination writers must strive to create fair, valid, and reliable examinations. Writing MCQs that assess higher-ordered thinking is difficult but possible by following specific guidelines, and especially by ensuring that the item writers are competent in their field.[16] Several evidence-based principles of preparing effective and objective tests are listed in the literature.[17]

Clarity, testing a broad range of topics, and consistency with content to be tested are vital for test makers to improve the fairness of examinations.[18] Well-thought learning objectives are pivotal to the creation of appropriate MCQs. A systematic approach starts with a detailed blueprint with outlines of the content to be tested and the expected level of examinee achievement in those areas.[19,20] The examination agency must provide the learning objectives to be assessed and content outlines to the writers before they start writing questions. MCQs must map to their corresponding learning outcomes.[21]

Question writers should be familiar with two qualifiers when assessing a question's quality: difficulty and discrimination. Difficulty refers to the percentage of students who will answer the question correctly. Discrimination refers to an MCQ's ability to differentiate between test takers who know the material versus those who do not.[6] Writers should limit introducing "irrelevant difficulty" and "test-wiseness." The irrelevant difficulty is the increase in the question's difficulty due to the introduction of flaws contrary to standard writing practices. It is essential to minimize the introduction of errors such as word cues, grammatical cues, longer correct answers, absolute terms, and convergence that test-wise candidates can use to answer the questions.[1,22]

Questions that do not follow the standard multiple-choice item-writing guidelines have low reliability and validity and may introduce construct-irrelevant variance (CIV) into testing.[23] CIV refers to extraneous variables that include poor question design that can affect the validity of assessment outcomes.[24] This phenomenon is especially pertinent to students with lower reading comprehension or who speak English as a second language.[25] Emulating the writing standards for MCQs is a critical way to reduce the introduction of construct-irrelevant variance and test-wiseness that may impact the reliability and validity of these tests. Reviewing of questions in a committee review improves their quality.[26] Editing MCQs based on best practices improves item clarity and substantially increases their performance.[27]

QUALITIES OF GOOD QUESTIONS

Single best response questions have a stem and response options, one of which is the key or the correct answer, while the others are distractors. **Fig. 1** lays down the rubric of a single best response MCQ. Alternately, there are questions known as K-style questions that may have multiple correct responses. This article focuses on single best response questions.

A high-quality MCQ usually takes about an hour to write, so authors should be cautious about apportioning requisite time, as time crunch can introduce irreparable item flaws due to overlooking standard practices. Questions should test core concepts and knowledge required to assess competence in specific domains versus testing "zebra" diagnoses or obscure facts. Good questions can be read, interpreted, and analyzed in their allotted time to yield an unambiguously clear answer. They have focused stems and options that are concise, plausible, mutually exclusive, free from clues, and do not contain "all of the above" or "none of the above."[2]

Questions must be appropriate for the level of training, be defensible, and supported by high-quality, unambiguous references. Test writers should avoid excessive verbosity; otherwise, the question becomes a test of reading speed and comprehension versus knowledge assessment. Importantly, good-quality MCQs have a high discrimination index and can differentiate between those who know the content and those who do not. A discrimination index above 0.2 is preferred, with the higher number indicating a greater validity of the question. Creating high-quality MCQs that test complex thinking versus fact-based recall requires time, training, and practice. Breaches of standard multiple-choice test writing guidelines are known as Item-Writing Flaws (IWFs). Test-wise examinees can discern cues in the item or options that can help them pick the right choices. Thus, test construction deficiencies may reward examinees with superior test-taking skills rather than knowledge of the content tested.[22]

The A–Z list of multiple-choice question writing tips in **Box 1** synthesizes several well-established standards.

WRITING GOOD STEMS

Writing good stems is essential for writing high-quality questions. The stem must be meaningful, relevant, and avoid negative statements.[2] The basic rule of writing the stem is that the question should be understandable without reading it multiple times and without reading all the options.[36]

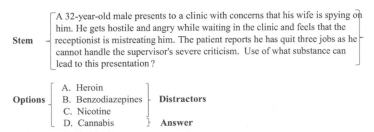

(S-Stem, O-Options, D-Distractors, A-Answer, Mnemonic-SODA)

Stem — A 32-year-old male presents to a clinic with concerns that his wife is spying on him. He gets hostile and angry while waiting in the clinic and feels that the receptionist is mistreating him. The patient reports he has quit three jobs as he cannot handle the supervisor's severe criticism. Use of what substance can lead to this presentation?

Options
A. Heroin
B. Benzodiazepines — **Distractors**
C. Nicotine
D. Cannabis — **Answer**

Fig. 1. The rubric of a single response multiple-choice question.

Box 1
A–Z of creating high-quality multiple-choice questions

A: Avoid cues, and clues

B: Biased and stereotyped language must be avoided

C: Cultural bias should be limited by avoiding slang, idioms, or colloquialisms

D: Distractors should be plausible and homogeneous in content, detail, and grammar

E: Effective use of language with correct grammar

F: Focused stems that include the central idea

G: Gender-neutral language should be used

H: "Hand test" must be passed*

I: Independent of vague quantifiers such as "usually," "mostly," and "rarely"

J: Joining multiple questions or concepts (double-barreled questions) is not recommended

K: Knowledge tested should be "important" and appropriate for the level of training

L: Length of distractors should be similar

M: Mutually exclusive and nonoverlapping distractors

N: "None of the above" and "all of the above" should not be used as distractors

O: One construct/point should be tested at a time

P: Positively worded stems should be used; avoid negative wording like "not" or "except"

Q: Question format is preferred compared with sentence completion

R: Reduce cognitive load for test-takers to be able to read, analyze and answer in time

S: Supported by data or references

T: Test higher-order learning

U: Unambiguous best answer unless using multiple correct response type questions

V: Vocabulary used should be simple for the test to measure knowledge versus reading

W: Window dressing or excessive verbosity should be avoided

X: X-factor(standout) or contradictory distractors should not be used

Y: Yearly posttest analysis

Z: Zebra diagnoses should be avoided

*Hand Test:

1 The examinee should be able to cover up the answers and answer by reading the stem only.

2 When writing vignettes, the test writer should cover up the stem except for the lead-in to make sure the vignette is necessary.

* The MCQs should pass Test 1, and MCQ vignettes should pass both 1 and 2".

Data from Refs.[2,17,19,25,28–35]

Quintessentially, the test of a good stem is whether or not a student who knows the material being tested can read the stem, cover up the answer choices (the "hand test"), and correctly answer the question. For that to occur, the stem must be focused and contain the bulk of the content. When writing questions, test writers should ensure that they pass the "hand test" to provide a focused stem.

What is true of the side effects of lithium?

In this example, a test-taker knowledgeable about lithium's side effects can generate many responses, not just about the side effects themselves, but also of aspects of those side effects. For the same reason, questions using NOT, LEAST, and EXCEPT do not conform to good-quality MCQ standards, as the range of possible answers can be infinite, and thus, the item cannot pass the hand test. The test-taker now must examine each answer choice and apply a true/false evaluation. Published literature on writing clinical scenario questions has posited that lead-ins should start with "what" instead of "which of the following" because the latter requires the examinee to know the specific answer choices, thereby lessening the effectiveness of the hand test.[37]

To make the stem focused, select an objective for the question, and then construct it to test that point specifically.

What medication is the best initial option to treat lithium-induced tremor?

Questions should test only one point at a time. It is easy to write a double-barreled question mistakenly and to spot one by looking for a conjunction in the lead-in.

What psychotherapy modality requires a thought journal and evaluation of automatic thoughts?

If a test-taker knows the answer to either part of the lead-in, they are not required to know the other part. To rework a double-barreled question as this, remove one part of the question.

What psychotherapy modality requires an evaluation of automatic thoughts?

Although it is not fair for questions to be "tricky," it is reasonable for questions to be difficult. A good test should have a range of easy, medium, and challenging questions to discriminate between test-takers adequately. A test question can require the examinee to go through several thought levels or steps to generate the answer. Deeper-level items can be created using a clinical scenario.

A 30-year-old man, who has a 10-year history of schizophrenia, is hospitalized for the eighth time in 2 years due to the exacerbation of command auditory hallucinations and paranoia. His past medications include haloperidol, olanzapine, risperidone, aripiprazole, perphenazine, quetiapine and the long-acting injections of haloperidol, paliperidone, and risperidone. The previous treatments did not improve the patient's symptoms significantly. The patient lives with his parents, who inform the physician, "We will do whatever it takes to get our son well." The patient states, "Give me any medication that will help."

First-level question lead-in: *What medication should the physician recommend to start next?*

Second-level question lead-in: *What is the most concerning side effect of the medication that should be started?*

NOT/EXCEPT/LEAST questions are among the quickest to write because of the ease of coming up with only 1 wrong answer when multiple right answers are available rather than creating 4 plausible distractors.

What antidepressant should NOT be the first-line therapy for a patient with a newly diagnosed major depressive disorder who has never been on medication?

Writing the options for the preceding question is a simple task for the test writer. List 4 selective serotonin reuptake inhibitors (SSRIs) and any non-SSRI. The question is complete! However, the preceding question stem is flawed for several reasons previously mentioned, and negatively phrased questions violate standard MCQ writing standards.

To fix this and several negatively phrased lead-ins without revising the rest of the stem, choose 1 SSRI as the correct answer, leave the non-SSRI as a distractor, devise 3 more distractors, and change the lead-in to read

What antidepressant should be the first-line therapy for a patient with a newly diagnosed major depressive disorder who has never been on medication?

VIGNETTES

In medical education, there is an increasing focus on testing higher-order skills and complex thinking. Clinical vignettes allow for testing the application of knowledge. They rely on sketches of patient history or other clinical information and often require medical decision making similar to making clinical decisions in real-world clinical practice. Hence, clinical vignettes are the preferred assessment format for several medical licensing and in-service training examinations. The US Medical Licensing Examination, used for assessing MD medical students and residents, uses vignettes for all test items, as vignettes require test-takers to demonstrate interpretation and problem solving instead of recall.[22]

A major pitfall in writing vignettes is a scenario that is irrelevant and not needed to answer the question. This extraneous information is known as "window dressing."

A 19-year-old man is brought to the emergency department by ambulance after he was seen by passers-by yelling at a statue in the park, telling it that he is Jesus. When approached by public safety officers, he said to them that they were the devil and told them, "I am sending you to hell." After extensive collaborative history and workup, he is diagnosed with new-onset schizophrenia. The emergency medicine physician would order which laboratory tests before starting an atypical antipsychotic?

In this example, the test-taker can answer the question using only the lead-in "The emergency medicine physician would order..." The preceding stem is extraneous. Much like a test-taker can use the hand test to cover up the answers, a question-writer can use the hand test to cover up all of the stem except for the lead-in to make sure the vignette is necessary. Furthermore, because clinical vignettes often test higher-order skills using complex thought processing, the time designated for testing should factor in the reading, thinking, and analysis required to answer clinical vignettes.

DISTRACTORS

Writing distractors is an art and is as important as writing a high-quality stem. Distractors should limit the ability of examinees to guess the correct answer. They should be plausible, clear, homogeneous, free from clues, not include "all of the above" or "none of the above," have the grammar consistent with the stem, and be parallel in form, similar in length, and use identical language.[17,28]

Bupropion works primarily for depression by blocking the reuptake of which of the following neurotransmitters?

A. Serotonin and Dopamine

B. Norepinephrine and Dopamine*
C. Norepinephrine and Histamine
D. Norepinephrine and acetylcholine
E. GABA and Dopamine

In this question, the astute test-taker will notice that Dopamine and norepinephrine occur more frequently as answer choices and assume that the answer featuring them is the correct answer using the *convergence* strategy. Other flaws include that the distractors are overlapping and not mutually exclusive.

A 35-year-old man visited the fertility clinic with his wife, as the couple wishes to have a child. He then has a follow-up visit with his psychiatrist for opioid dependence and is started on maintenance treatment with methadone. Which of the following is an adverse effect of this treatment?

A. Hypogonadism*
B. Hypergonadism
C. Hyperglycemia
D. Hypertension
E. Hypothyroidism

In this question, the test-wise examinee will pick up the stem's cues and discern that answers A and B are opposites and narrow down the possible answer to a 50 to 50 guess. Thus, distractors should not contradict each other.

A 27-year-old patient has had a dysphoric mood, low energy, difficulty focusing, a 15-pound weight loss, and no interest in daily activities for more than 2 months. The patient has been taking fluoxetine regularly for 5 weeks without any improvement. Which of the following would be appropriate as the next step for management?

A. Labs for TSH and T4 to rule out hypothyroidism
B. Switch SSRI
C. Cognitive-behavioral therapy
D. Family history
E. SSRI and CBT
F. All of the above

The preceding question has several flaws with its distractors. Options are not homogeneous: A is about laboratory tests, B is about medication, C is about psychotherapy, D is about family history, E is a combination of medication and psychotherapy, and F is all the above. Option A is longer than other distractors. Options B and E, and C and E are overlapping and not mutually exclusive. Option D is not consistent with the lead-in statement, which asks for the next step in management. Other distractor flaws include no single correct answer, and "All of the above" is listed as a distractor.

A good or performing distractor is an option that is selected by at least 5% or more examinees as a possible answer.[38] The most significant improvement in MCQ performance is associated with the effective elimination of nonperforming distractors selected by a few test-takers.[27]

ITEM ANALYSIS

One way to analyze the quality of the questions and remove poor performers is through an item analysis post-examination. Items that have weak discriminatory power should be removed or replaced.[38]

The following are some terms commonly used in item analysis.

Difficulty index (p): This index refers to the percentage of students who correctly answered the question.

For example, if 70% of students correctly answered the question, the difficulty index (p) would be 0.70.

Extreme scores on the difficulty index can inform the writers about the quality of the question and whether it is working effectively as a discriminator of student knowledge or can be used in future examinations. Examinations should have items that vary across a range of difficulty.

Item discriminator index (d): This index is a measure of how well an item differentiates between low-performing and high-performing students, usually the top 25% and the bottom 25%.[22,29] d ranges from -1 to $+1$. Values >0.4 are considered good.[39] In general, an index score above 0.15 is usually acceptable. However, a larger number is preferable in separating between examinees who know the content versus those who do not. Highly discriminating items tend to lead to high score reliability.[23]

Another way to measure discrimination between items is the point-biserial correlation, which is the correlation between the right and wrong scores students receive on a question and the total score that the students receive as an aggregate on all the questions. Point-biserial values range from -1.0 to $+1.0$. A large positive point-biserial indicates that the item is a good discriminator. It means that examinees with high scores on the test answered the item correctly, and those with low scores did not. A low point-biserial indicates that the item is a poor discriminator, as the examinees who received low scores on the test answered the item correctly, whereas the examinees who received a high score on the test got the item wrong.[40]

Posttest analysis for difficult questions includes checking the right answer and substituting a confusing acceptor. This analysis also involves removing the question because of lack of clarity, low discrimination, overlapping objectives with other items, or a preponderance of difficult questions.[41] Fewer than 5% of test-takers choose nonfunctioning distractors, and they should be revised or removed to improve the quality of questions.[42] Multiple-choice examination writers should consider the guidelines in **Table 1** but avoid setting any hard cutoffs to remove items.[43] Item statistics and item analysis are essential to maintain quality control, decrease item flaws, and help improve the quality of future examinations.[44]

Table 1
Multiple-choice questions: glossary of terms

Multiple-choice question/Item	A statement with a problem to be solved or a question to be answered based on available options
Stem	Problem or question based on learning objectives
Option	A possible answer to the stem
Distractor	An incorrect answer
Answer	Correct answer among options and is also known as the key
Learning objectives	Learning goals of the assessment
Item-writing flaw (IWF)	Violation of multiple-choice question/Item-writing guidelines

DISCUSSION

MCQs are the most common form of standardized testing available in medical education and psychiatry. Guidelines based on evidence and experience help guide writing MCQs. Less-experienced item writers should first familiarize themselves with the terms and concepts in **Table 2**. The A–Z recommendations in **Box 1** are a synthesis of the best MCQ writing practices from several published guidelines. It may not be feasible to test certain content areas using the rubric suggested in these guidelines. Flexibility is recommended for testing knowledge in content areas in which it is not easy to write higher-order questions (eg, normal child development). Examination writers must perform a posttest item analysis after becoming familiar with the terms that indicate a specific question's performance and learning the application of statistical results to posttest item analysis and review. The parameters laid out in **Table 3** and other literature on the posttest item analysis may be helpful. Posttest item analysis and peer review play a vital role in improving the quality of future examinations.

Practice and experience writing multiple test items with peer feedback lead to improvements in writing MCQs. Question writers should continually screen the questions they write to conform to the best-practice standards listed in **Box 1**. Post-tests, peer review committees must assess the quality and effectiveness of MCQs as reliable and valid test items.

Standardized testing will continue to rely on multiple-choice tests in the future for a plethora of advantages they offer over other conventional assessment methods.

Table 2 Statistics and posttest item analysis	
Validity	Degree to which the multiple-choice test measures examinee knowledge.
Reliability	Degree to which the multiple-choice test produces similar results if the test is repeated.
Construct-irrelevant variance	The systematic error introduced by variables unrelated to the construct being measured that affects the accuracy and validity of results.
Item analysis	Provides data on the quality and effectiveness of a specific test item.
Difficulty index or item difficulty (p)	Percentage of examinees who answered a particular item correctly. Ranges from 0 to 1. Higher values denote an easier question.
Item discriminator index (d)	The measure of how well an item differentiates between low-performing and high-performing examinees. Low performers are usually in the bottom 25th percentile, and high performers are usually in the top 25th percentile. Ranges from −1.0 to +1.0.
Point-biserial correlation	Measures how well a question discriminates between examinees with higher knowledge and lower knowledge by responses to a specific question and scores on the overall test. Positive if higher scorers answered the question correctly than lower performers and negative if the opposite occurred. Ranges from −1.0 to +1.0.

Analysis Glossary of Terms.
  Data from Refs.[22,24,25,45–47]

Table 3
Recommendations based on difficulty and discrimination indices

Difficulty (p)	Discrimination (d)	Interpretation	Action
<0.60	<0.15	Difficult item with poor discrimination	Consider removing item
<0.60	≥0.15	Difficult item with high discrimination	Retain item
0.60–0.90	≤0	Moderate to low-difficulty item with negative discrimination	Consider removing item
0.60–0.90	0 < d < 0.15	Moderate to low-difficulty item with low discrimination	Retain but consider revising for future tests
0.60–0.90	>0.15	Moderate to low-difficulty item with high discrimination	Retain, this is the ideal score range in which most questions should be located
>.90	Disregard	Low-difficulty item	If retaining, consider revising for future tests

Adapted from Rudolph M, Daugherty K, Ray M, Shuford V, Lebovitz L, Di Vall M. Best Practices Related to Examination Item Construction and Post-hoc Review. Am J Pharm Educ. 2019;83(7):7204.

However, they have their shortcomings, which impede the quality of the assessment process. Educators in psychiatry and medical education should continue to practice and advance best practices in multiple-choice test creation to provide valid assessments. As research shows, high-quality MCQs are effective learning as well as assessment tools. Using the best practices in their composition can significantly impact medical education and assessment.

SUMMARY

Well-constructed, peer-reviewed MCQs meet the several requirements of good-quality assessments besides lower cost and ease of administration.[48] Clarity of testing objectives, familiarity, and practice with test writing guidelines, understanding item analysis, and improving examination reliability and validity are critical to writing high-quality MCQs.[25] Creating high-quality MCQs and eliminating faulty items enhances the validity of standardized tests and is important for fair and objective assessments. Hence, faculty and item writers entrusted with creating multiple-choice tests must familiarize themselves with the established best-practice standards to write high-quality MCQs for examinees that nullify the effects of extraneous variables. Regular training, practice, and peer feedback with item analysis post-testing can be useful tools for improving the quality of MCQs.

DISCLOSURE

The authors have no financial disclosures.

REFERENCES

1. Coughlin P, Featherstone C. How to write a high quality multiple-choice question (MCQ): a guide for clinicians. Eur J Vasc Endovasc Surg 2017;54(5):654–8.

2. Salam A, Yousuf R, Bakar S. Multiple-choice questions in medical education: how to construct high quality questions. Int J Hum Health Sci 2020;4(2):79.
3. Bontis N, Hardie T, Serenko A. Techniques for assessing skills and knowledge in a business strategy classroom. Int J Teach Case Stud 2009;2(2):162–80.
4. Anderson L, Krathwohl D. A taxonomy for learning, teaching, and assessing: a revision of bloom's taxonomy of educational objectives. 1st edition. New York: Longman; 2001.
5. Little J, Bjork E. Optimizing multiple-choice tests as tools for learning. Mem Cognit 2014;43(1):14–26.
6. Boland R, Lester N, Williams E. Writing multiple-choice questions. Acad Psychiatry 2010;34(4):310–6.
7. Melnick D, Dillon G, Swanson D. Medical licensing examinations in the United States. J Dent Educ 2002;66(5):595–9.
8. Webb E, Phuong J, Naeger D. Does educator training or experience affect the quality of multiple-choice questions? Acad Radiol 2015;22(10):1317–22.
9. Nedeau-Cayo R, Laughlin D, Rus L, et al. Assessment of item-writing flaws in multiple-choice questions. J Nurses Prof Dev 2013;29(2):52–7.
10. Breakall J, Randles C, Tasker R. Development and use of a multiple-choice item writing flaws evaluation instrument in the context of general chemistry. Chem Educ Res Pract 2019;20(2):369–82.
11. Pais J, Silva A, Guimarães B, et al. Do item-writing flaws reduce examinations psychometric quality? BMC Res Notes 2016;9(1):399.
12. Pate A, Caldwell D. Effects of multiple-choice item-writing guideline utilization on item and student performance. Currents Pharm Teach Learn 2014;6(1):130–4.
13. Capan Melser M, Steiner-Hofbauer V, Lilaj B, et al. Knowledge, application and how about competence? Qualitative assessment of multiple-choice questions for dental students. Med Educ Online 2020;25(1):1714199.
14. Pham H, Besanko J, Devitt P. Examining the impact of specific types of item-writing flaws on student performance and psychometric properties of the multiple-choice question. McdEdPublish 2018;7(4).
15. Khan H, Danish K, Awan A, et al. Identification of technical item flaws leads to improvement of the quality of single best multiple-choice questions. Pak J Med Sci 2013;29(3):715–8.
16. Downing S, Haladyna T. Handbook of test development. Mahwah, NJ: L. Erlbaum; 2006.
17. Haladyna T, Downing S, Rodriguez M. A review of multiple-choice item-writing guidelines for classroom assessment. Appl Meas Educ 2002;15(3):309–33.
18. McCoubrie P. Improving the fairness of multiple-choice questions: a literature review. Med Teach 2004;26(8):709–12.
19. Ray M, Daugherty K, Lebovitz L, et al. Best practices on examination construction, administration, and feedback. Am J Pharm Educ 2018;82(10):7066.
20. Sutherland K, Schwartz J, Dickison P. Best practices for writing test items. J Nurs Regul 2012;3(2):35–9.
21. Collins J. Writing multiple-choice questions for continuing medical education activities and self-assessment modules. Radiographics 2006;26(2):543–51.
22. Paniagua M, Swygert K. Constructing written test questions for the basic and clinical Sciences. 4th edition 2016. Available at: https://www.nbme.org/sites/default/files/2020-01/IWW_Gold_Book.pdf. Accessed July 18, 2020.
23. Downing S. The effects of violating standard item writing principles on tests and students: the consequences of using flawed test items on achievement examinations in medical education. Adv Health Sci Educ Theory Pract 2005;10(2):133–43.

24. Haladyna T, Downing S. Construct-irrelevant variance in high-stakes testing. Educ Meas Issues Pract 2005;23(1):17–27.
25. Rudolph M, Daugherty K, Ray M, et al. Best practices related to examination item construction and post-hoc review. Am J Pharm Educ 2019;83(7):7204.
26. Wallach P, Crespo L, Holtzman K, et al. Use of a committee review process to improve the quality of course examinations. Adv Health Sci Educ 2006; 11(1):61–8.
27. Bertoni F, Smales L, Trent B, et al. Do item writing best practices improve multiple-choice questions for university students? Journal of Financial Education 2019;45(2).
28. Haladyna T, Downing S. A taxonomy of multiple-choice item-writing rules. Appl Meas Educ 1989;2(1):37–50.
29. Lane S, Raymond MR, Haladyna TM. Handbook of test development (educational psychology handbook). 2nd edition. New York, NY: Routledge; 2015.
30. Brame C. Writing good multiple-choice test questions. Vanderbilt University; 2020. Availble at: https://cft.vanderbilt.edu/guides-sub-pages/writing-good-multiple-choice-test-questions/. Accessed July 21, 2020.
31. Frey B, Petersen S, Edwards L, et al. Item-writing rules: collective wisdom. Teach Teach Educ 2005;21(4):357–64.
32. Haladyna T, Downing S. Validity of a taxonomy of multiple-choice item-writing rules. Appl Meas Educ 1989;2(1):51–78.
33. DiBattista D, Sinnige-Egger J, Fortuna G. The "None of the Above" option in multiple-choice testing: an experimental study. J Exp Educ 2013;82(2):168–83.
34. Burton S, Sudweeks R, Merrill P, et al. How to prepare better multiple-choice test items: guidelines for University faculty 1991. Testing.byu.edu. Availble at: https://testing.byu.edu/handbooks/betteritems.pdf. Accessed July 21, 2020.
35. Dell K, Wantuch G. How-to-guide for writing multiple-choice questions for the pharmacy instructor. Currents Pharm Teach Learn 2017;9(1):137–44.
36. Chaudhary N, Bhatia B, Mahato S, et al. Multiple-choice questions-Part II (Classification, Item Preparation, Analysis and Banking). J Universal Coll Med Sci 2014;2(3):54–9.
37. Smith P, Mucklow J. Writing clinical scenarios for clinical science questions. Clin Med 2016;16(2):142–5.
38. DiBattista D, Kurzawa L. Examination of the quality of multiple-choice items on classroom tests. Can J Scholarship Teach Learn 2011;2(2).
39. Clifton S, Schriner C. Assessing the quality of multiple-choice test items. Nurse Educ 2010;35(1):12–6.
40. Varma S. Preliminary item statistics using point-biserial correlation and P-values, education data system. California: Morgan Hill; 2015. Jcesom.marshall.edu. Availble at: https://jcesom.marshall.edu/media/24104/Item-Stats-Point-Biserial.pdf. Accessed August 4, 2020.
41. Dory V, Allan K, Birnbaum L, et al. Ensuring the quality of multiple-choice tests. Acad Med 2019;94(5):740.
42. Gajjar S, Sharma R, Kumar P, et al. Item and test analysis to identify quality multiple-choice questions (MCQs) from an assessment of medical students of Ahmedabad, Gujarat. Indian J Community Med 2014;39(1):17–20.
43. Frey BB. Sage Encyclopedia of educational research, Measurement, and evaluation. Thousand Oaks, CA: Sage; 2018.
44. Xu X, Kauer S, Tupy S. Multiple-choice questions: tips for optimizing assessment in-seat and online. Scholarsh Teach Learn Psychol 2016;2(2):147–58.

45. Smith L. How to write better multiple-choice questions. Nursing 2018; 48(11):14–7.
46. Rauschert E, Yang S, Pigg R. Which of the following is true: we can write better multiple-choice questions. Bull Ecol Soc Am 2018;100(1):e01468.
47. Zimmaro D. Writing multiple-choice questions. Faculty Innovation Center; 2020. Availble at: https://facultyinnovate.utexas.edu/multiple-choice-questions. Accessed July 21, 2020.
48. Palmer E, Devitt P. Assessment of higher order cognitive skills in undergraduate education: modified essay or multiple-choice questions? Research paper. BMC Med Educ 2007;7(1):49.

Finding the Story in Medicine

The Use of Narrative Techniques in Psychiatry

Elizabeth Fenstermacher, MD[a,b,*], Regina M. Longley, BA[c],
Hermioni L. Amonoo, MD, MPP[d,e,f]

KEYWORDS

- Narrative medicine • Curriculum • Empathy • Graduate medical education
- Internship and residency • Education models • Health personnel education

KEY POINTS

- There are 12 principles of adult learning.
- Narrative medicine techniques leverage principles of adult learning.
- Narrative medicine has an established andragogy that is versatile and allows for structured application across many narrative forms.
- Narrative medicine offers unique benefit to psychiatry by facilitating empathic connection and exploration of countertransference.

INTRODUCTION

Learning requires understanding. Yet, the vast body of current medical knowledge requires that medical students and trainees learn more within an ever-shrinking and overdetermined didactic schedule. Thus, medical educators now face the formidable task of fitting expansive medical knowledge into a foreshortened time frame while maintaining a comprehensible human framework.

This article explores how narrative medicine may ameliorate this predicament by optimizing adult learning while also offering unique humanistic benefit; this is accomplished by considering the following: (1) principles of adult learning, (2) how narrative medicine appears to uniquely leverage adult learning principles, and (3) the evidence

[a] Department of Psychiatry, Denver Health, 660 Bannock St, Suite 4754, Denver, CO 80204, USA;
[b] University of Colorado, School of Medicine, 13001 E 17th Pl, Aurora, CO 80045, USA;
[c] Department of Psychiatry, Massachusetts General Hospital, 125 Nashua Street, Suite #324, Boston, MA 02114, USA; [d] Harvard Medical School, 25 Shattuck Street, Boston, MA 02115, USA;
[e] Department of Psychiatry, Brigham and Women's Hospital, 60 Fenwood Road, 4th Floor, Boston, MA 02115, USA; [f] Department of Psychosocial Oncology, Dana-Farber Cancer Institute, 450 Brookline Avenue, Boston, MA 02215, USA
* Corresponding author. Cambridge Hospital, Department of Child Psychiatry, 1493 Cambridge Street, Cambridge, MA 02139.
E-mail address: elizabeth.fenstermacher@dhha.org

Psychiatr Clin N Am 44 (2021) 263–281
https://doi.org/10.1016/j.psc.2021.03.006
0193-953X/21/© 2021 Elsevier Inc. All rights reserved.

psych.theclinics.com

base for use of narratives in medical education, (4) the particular promise of narrative medicine within psychiatry (5) a proposed model narrative medicine curriculum for a 4-year psychiatric residency training program.

PRINCIPLES OF ADULT LEARNING

Although innate learning processes underly learning across the life span, educating adults poses unique advantages and challenges.[1–3] Adults are self-directed learners who critically appraise learning opportunities before engaging with them.[1–3] Consequently, motivation is crucial to adult learning.[1,2] The central importance of both engaging adult learners and utilizing adult learning principles to the success of adult learning initiatives has been demonstrated in tasks that vary from creating patient educational brochures to designing a residency curriculum.[1,2]

Modern andragogy—the study of adult learning—describes significant differences between adult learners and child learners.[4] Developed in the mid-twentieth century by Malcolm Knowles, modern andragogy offers key assumptions that promote optimal adult learning.[4] Expanding on Knowles' work, Jane Vella[3] identified 12 core principles that foster adult learning and establish its necessary preconditions.[3] **Table 1** summarizes Vella's principles.

Table 1 Principles of adult learning	
Principle	**Description**
1. Needs assessment	Define learners' expectations, current knowledge, learning needs/wants.
2. Safety	Adults need psychological safety to learn.
3. Sound relationships	Friendship between the teacher and learners, based on mutuality without dependency
4. Sequence/reinforcement	Material presented coherently in sequence (eg, easy → hard) with frequent opportunities for reinforcement
5. Praxis	Action with reflection or learning by doing
6. Respect for learners	Respecting learners as decision makers, the subjects of learning
7. Ideas, feelings, actions	Incorporation of cognitive, affective, and psychomotor aspects of learning
8. Immediacy	Perceived immediate usefulness, related to learner's context
9. Role development	Equity between teachers and students. Students are not passive recipients of information but engaged in dialogic discussion.
10. Teamwork	The assurance of safety and shared responsibility within teams facilitate adult learning.
11. Engagement	Learning is viewed as a fundamentally participative process, dependent on learner engagement.
12. Accountability	Who is accountable to whom? Adult learners are accountable to themselves and teachers; teachers are accountable to their students.

Data from: Vella JK. *Learning to Listen, Learning to Teach : the Power of Dialogue in Educating Adults.* San Francisco: Jossey-Bass; 2002.

Knowles' and Vella's work highlights that the foundational task of educating adult learners is to create a curriculum and environment that motivate and facilitate self-directed learning.[3,4] Although an unengaged learner will not succeed, a learner in a learning environment that does not emphasize relevant content, effective learning strategies, and a culture of safety will experience diminished returns. Vella's emphasis on safety and the learning environment underscores the importance that learning theory places on both social context and emotional state of the learner in the learning process. It also provides actionable guidance on how to optimize these to promote learning.[5-7]

Vella's principles of adult learning are dependent on one another, and she identifies many links in her work.[3] In this article, these principles are simplified into 3 core categories (relevance, efficacy, and environment). Relevance encompasses those elements of Vella's principles that demonstrate that the learning task has applicability to adult learners' needs and are relevant to their current or future learning goals. Efficacy encapsulates core educational techniques that Vella has identified as particularly salient to adult learners. These techniques are widely recognized as effective and efficient, which is important to engaging adult learners who may reject less-efficient or lower-yield curricula, particularly if there is a perception of a high time cost burden.[3] Environment captures the importance of creating a space where adult learners allow for the vulnerability inherent in learning.

Fig. 1 depicts Vella's principles of adult learning organized by these core categories. The authors have suggested which principles fit within these core categories and which fit into areas of overlap. relevance (1. needs assessment and 8. immediacy), efficacy (4. sequence/reinforcement, 5. praxis, and 10. teamwork), and environment (2. safety, 3. sound relationships, and 6. respect for learners). Note the areas of overlap

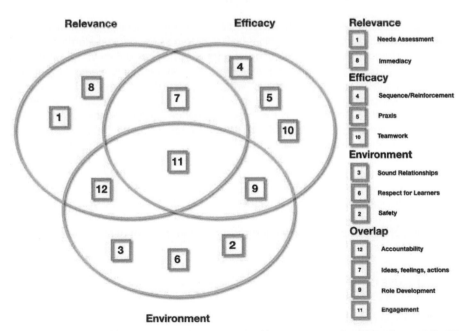

Fig. 1. Vella's principles of adult learning organized by core categories. (*Data from*: Vella JK. *Learning to Listen, Learning to Teach : the Power of Dialogue in Educating Adults.* San Francisco: Jossey-Bass; 2002.)

between these core categories include (7. ideas/feelings/actions, 9. clear roles and role development, and 12. accountability). The eleventh principle, engagement, is complex and depends not only on individual factors (emotional state and prior experiences) but also on an adult learner's appraisal of how well the curricula meets their learning needs and social context.[3,5-7]

NARRATIVE MEDICINE DEFINED

Narrative medicine is a structured, patient-centered approach that seeks to promote humanistic engagement of medical practitioners through the application of narrative.[8,9] This is accomplished practically through *attending*, *representing*, and *affiliating*.[9] *Attending* refers to perceptive attention,[9] a process in which close scrutiny and careful attention allow a learner to perceive what is being presented.[9] *Representing* refers to the process of capturing or conferring one's perception into a material representation; by creating a material representation of one's thoughts, these thoughts are made more evident to both self and others.[9] *Affiliating* refers to the increased sense of connection and unity accomplished through increased empathy and understanding. By accomplishing and generalizing the tasks of narrative medicine, attending, representing, affiliating, a provider can be more fully present with their patients and colleagues (attend), hold a clearer mental understanding and picture of their patient's experiences (represent), and connect emotionally with their patients and colleagues (affiliate).[9] Narrative medicine offers a unique framework for understanding medical encounters for both the patient and the physician.[8]

THE ANDRAGOGY OF NARRATIVE MEDICINE

Milota and colleagues[10] recently reviewed the current evidence for narrative medicine and identified 3 core andragogical (referred to as pedagogical elements in their writing; andragogy is used in this article for internal consistency) elements that accomplish attending, representing, affiliating. The andragogical elements identified include reading-reflecting-responding, which the authors define as (1) reading— reflective engagement with a primary source (often a patient narrative); (2) reflecting—a personal reflection about the first experience (often a written assignment); and (3) responding—sharing and discussing.[10] By identification of these 3 core elements of narrative medicine, Milota and colleagues[10] offer a systematic andragogical approach to the practice of narrative medicine.

Although such a systematic methodology is valuable to the implementation of narrative medicine and standardization of curricula to promote dissemination, it can portray narrative medicine as a series of sterilized steps. At its core, narrative medicine concerns itself with the highest ideals of medicine and, arguably, of humanity itself—the promotion of true empathic connection through enhancement of skills in observation, listening, and reflecting.

HOW THE USE OF NARRATIVE DIRECTLY INCORPORATES ADULT LEARNING PRINCIPLES INTO MEDICAL EDUCATION

The 3 core andragogical components of narrative medicine (close reading, self-reflection, and discussion) align with Vella's adult learning principles.[3,9,10] How the 3 core components of narrative medicine synergistically promote adult learning is discussed.

Close Reading

Close reading of a narrative captures the learner's attention amidst recall and association of individual past experiences; it aids associative learning and fulfills Vella's principles of engagement, immediacy, and needs assessment.[3,11] By engaging with a narrative, the reader is propelled into a state of curiosity. Within the reader, immediacy arises from the need to understand the author's perspective, and the gap in understanding between the reader and the author provides a natural and intrinsic needs assessment.

Self-Reflection

The process of reflection further accomplishes Vella's principles of sound relationships, respect for learners, praxis, and ideas/feelings/actions.[3] The evocation of reflection affirms the learner as an equal partner in a hierarchical learning space. It accomplishes the goal of sound relationships by making it clear that the learner is viewed as having independent agency and demonstrates respect for learners. The process of reflection is itself a praxis, action with reflection, where the learner is propelled beyond passive experiential perceptions into an active evaluative space. Similarly, by creating a representation of their perceptions as part of the reflective process, learners simultaneously engage ideas/feelings/actions, thereby deepening self-understanding while accessing both their affective and cognitive responses.

Discussion

Open dialogue and collaborative discussion with peers and instructors again reinforce sound relationships and respect for learners but also elicits clear roles and role development, while enhancing teamwork and ensuring accountability.[3] Through dialogic discussion of close readings and reflections, the learner engages actively in education from the vantage point of human equality between teacher and students. This bidirectional engagement helps them to assume new roles as active dialogic participants fulfilling clear roles and role development. Teamwork is accomplished through the collaborative process of dialogic discourse and accountability is ensured through mutual responsibility to colearners and instructor.

The last of Vella's principles, safety and sequence/reinforcement, are embodied within all steps of narrative medicine, with considerable time and space in the literature devoted to the need for safety as a prerequisite.[3,8,9] The andragogy itself is embedded intrinsically in the idea of sequence/reinforcement, with learners first developing their own conceptualization through close reading and active reflection before experiencing the transfiguration of an idea within the vessel of social learning. The embedded social learning in narrative medicine elicits these intrinsic learning processes, which are active from early childhood.[6]

EXPANDING THE CONCEPT OF A NARRATIVE IN MEDICAL EDUCATION

The most common way a narrative is incorporated into medical education is through the use of a clinical vignette. Clinical vignettes offer easy and accessible ways to incorporate teaching points and highlight key diagnostic and treatment concerns. However, the use of "narrative" expands far beyond the clinical vignette.[8,9,12,13] Although formal narrative medicine interventions offer benefit to learners, it also is important to stress opportunities to leverage narrative outside a structured andragogy. Examples of narratives are provided in **Box 1** and can include reflective writing, evaluating a work of

> **Box 1**
> **Types of narrative within narrative medicine[8–10,12–18]**
>
> Clinical vignette
>
> Reflective writing
>
> Work of literary fiction
>
> Autobiographical patient perspective
>
> Artwork (print media)
>
> Musical piece
>
> Cinema film
>
> Performative theater
>
> Poetry
>
> Workshopping participants writing
>
> Online forum participation

literary fiction, workshopping a participant's writing, going to a museum, presenting a play, and even participating in online forums.[8–10,14,15]

EVIDENCE FOR THE USE OF NARRATIVE IN MEDICAL EDUCATION

Over the past 2 decades, narrative medicine programs have become widespread globally.[8–10,19] Narrative medicine has been demonstrated to be effective in promoting empathy, reflection, professionalism, and trustworthiness.[8,9] Increased empathy has been reported robustly.[8,9,12,14,19–21] Often measured by standardized self-report scales, these gains in empathy have been demonstrated across professional disciplines (medicine, nursing, dentistry, physical therapy, and nutrition), at all levels of training (from preprofessional training to postgraduate practice), within different cultural frameworks, and with a variety of narrative medicine design interventions (reflective writing, performance, and so forth).[12,14,19–21] Improvements in self-reflection appear to be mediated by changes in internal and external observational skills and include expansion of reflective skepticism, self-examination, and critical open mindedness.[22] Increases in self-reflection have been demonstrated to have a positive impact on clinical work, including enhanced incorporation of feedback, improved diagnostic accuracy in challenging cases, and expanded overall clinical reasoning.[10,18]

Narrative medicine also promotes communication and collaboration (eg, the patient-doctor relationship) in medicine.[8,10,12,14,15,17,23] Improvements in patient–health care provider communication via narrative medicine correlated with higher scores in trust, perception of physician receptivity, patient-centered information giving, rapport building, and facilitation of patient involvement factors.[8,9,22] Physician competence in narrative techniques also has been linked to improvements in various health outcomes (eg, reduced cancer pain, improved lung function in asthma, and improved immune response following hepatitis B immunization).[24]

The evidence for narrative medicine's impact on clinical knowledge and academic performance is still limited but promising. In a 2-year, prospective study, Yang and colleagues[21] investigated the impact of a narrative medicine intervention on 177 nursing students. They randomized participants to 3 groups: (1) a theoretical-only intervention group, (2) a combined theoretical and clinical practice intervention group, and (3) a control group. Both intervention groups had a statistically significant higher performance on overall internship scores than the control group.[21] Both intervention groups also had higher empathy scores, although this was only statistically significant for the combined group relative to controls.[21] Likewise, the combined intervention group had statistically significant higher thesis achievement compared with the control group, but the theoretical-only intervention group did not.[21] Similarly, Tsai and colleagues[17] demonstrated the impact of narrative medicine interventions on standardized testing. In a quasi-experimental, prospective study, they randomly selected 22 medical interns (from a class of 116) to participate in a narrative medicine training course.[17] Of those invited, 15 interns participated in a brief narrative course.[17] The year-end performance of those interns on the Objective Structured Clinical Examination (OSCE) then was compared with a control group of 39 nonparticipating interns matched by age, gender, and academic performance.[17] Following the single, brief narrative medicine course, participating interns had higher performance on the 2 OSCE stations focused on communication.[17]

THE APPLICATION OF NARRATIVE MEDICINE TO PSYCHIATRY

The direct application of narrative medicine in psychiatry has been limited. Narrative medicine, however, may offer particular benefit to psychiatric practitioners. Emphasizing the centrality of careful listening within a patient-physician encounter, narrative techniques enhance observational skills, self-reflection, and critical open-mindedness, which are foundational to psychiatric diagnosis and treatment.[22]

Moreover, narrative medicine offers a framework to explore counter-transferential feelings in psychiatric practice.[13] Deliberate listening in narrative medicine can allow for an exploration of hidden fears and helplessness.[16] Even more dramatically, an imagined autobiographical narrative can allow a direct examination of counter-transferential feelings within a treatment relationship, provide new treatment targets, and provide a clinician with clues about how to strengthen therapeutic alliance.[13,16,25]

Narrative techniques also may be a lens that allows exploration of stereotypes and stigma, which can lead medical students away from pursuing psychiatry as a specialty and may contribute to misdiagnosis.[25] Opportunities for discussion using narrative techniques and themes also allow residents to explore internalized assumptions and examine how societal and cultural factors influence psychiatric care.[26]

Although narrative medicine itself has not been adopted widely within psychiatric training and practice, narrative therapy techniques have been developed from the same tradition.[27] The goals of narrative therapy differ from those of narrative medicine in that the purpose is not empathic understanding but rather encouraging patients to collaboratively reframe their experience for therapeutic gain.[27] This different although similar tradition is highlighted to avoid confusion between narrative medicine and narrative therapy.

PROPOSAL OF A NARRATIVE MEDICINE CURRICULUM FOR PSYCHIATRY GRADUATE MEDICAL EDUCATION PROGRAMS

The versatility of narrative medicine across many narrative formats makes it broadly applicable to psychiatric graduate medical education programs.[8–10,12–18,26] The authors propose courses that build on the work of prior narrative medicine programs[9,13,26] for a comprehensive and longitudinal narrative medicine curriculum (**Table 2**) and a 4-year psychiatry residency program (**Table 3**).

Table 2
Sample individual narrative medicine courses for psychiatry graduate medical education programs

Proposed Courses	Description
Introduction to narrative techniques[9]	An instructor-led course on the principles and practice of narrative medicine
Becoming a psychiatrist[26]	An instructor-led course on key topics that inform the identity of a psychiatrist
Psychiatric diagnosis[26]	An instructor-led course on the meaning making of psychiatric labels and how the use of a diagnosis influences patients' perceptions of themselves as well as how they are viewed by others
Psychiatric treatment[26]	An instructor-led course on treatment approaches, with a focus on shifts in treatment modalities over time and societal context to help residents challenge their own assumptions about different psychiatric therapies
Illness experience[26]	An instructor-led course on individual patient experience of illness
Narrative supervision[13]	Weekly individual supervision with a faculty member who reads and reflects with a resident on narrative writing Residents can be encouraged to create an imagined autobiographical narrative which offers particular insight into the resident's counter-transferential feelings.
Peer discussion group, literature based[9]	A facilitated group discussion in which residents discuss their experiences with narrative medicine readings
Peer discussion group, case based[9,13]	A facilitated group discussion in which residents generate narratives from their own clinical experiences. These narratives could include imagined autobiographical narratives to allow for discussion of countertransference. This group should be offered only in the final years of residency, given the inherent vulnerability of this process and need for group cohesion and safety.
Narrative movie nights[9]	Viewing of a movie followed by a discussion of important thematic content as it pertains to narrative medicine. The group-based discussion could be either resident-led or faculty-led.

The authors' narrative medicine curriculum allows for gradual development and mastery of reading-reflecting-responding.[9] Following a brief introduction to narrative medicine—its origins and goals—the authors suggest immediately applying narrative techniques within a course on becoming a psychiatrist, because this leads to rapid internalization of the skills essential to narrative medicine.[9,26] This format would allow for the promotion of an early group identity for psychiatric residents through shared empathic reading. Residents then would practice these skills further via courses on psychiatric treatment and psychiatric diagnosis in their second year. As residents

Table 3	
Proposed narrative medicine curriculum for psychiatry residents	
Postgraduate Year	**Curriculum Elements**
PGY1	Introduction to narrative techniques (instructor-led course, 2 sessions)
	Becoming a psychiatrist (instructor-led course, 4 sessions)
	Optional, narrative movie nights (movie showing with faculty discussant, monthly)
PGY2	Individual narrative supervision (1 h supervision/week)
	Psychiatric diagnosis (instructor-led course, 4 sessions)
	Psychiatric treatment (instructor-led course, 7 sessions)
	Optional, narrative movie nights (movie showing with faculty discussant, monthly)
PGY3	Individual narrative supervision (1 h supervision/week)
	Peer discussion group, literature based (1 group/month)
	Optional, narrative movie nights (movie showing with faculty discussant, monthly)
PGY4	Illness experience (instructor-led course, 6 sessions)
	Elective, peer discussion group, case-based material
	Optional, individual narrative supervision
	Optional, narrative movie nights (movie showing with faculty discussant, monthly)

Abbreviation: PGY, postgraduate year.

gain more familiarity and expertise with narrative medicine in the first 2 years, they will be poised to provide narrative suggestions for development of their third-year curriculum. In addition to specific readings, the authors propose individual narrative supervision beginning in the second postgraduate year to allow for exploration of stigma, stereotypes, and countertransference within the safety of individual supervision. The curriculum is designed with vulnerability in mind to allow residents to establish a sense of group safety and cohesion prior to more vulnerable applications of narrative medicine like individual narrative supervision and case-based narrative groups. The authors strongly suggest that the advanced peer discussion group using case-based material be entirely elective for this purpose.

Appendix 1 provides specific recommendations for narratives, discussion questions, and homework for proposed courses that easily can be customized by training programs.

DISCUSSION

Narrative medicine as a field arose out of the need to promote humanistic engagement in medical fields where such connections were threatened by competing demands and time pressures. At its core, narrative medicine allows physicians to understand and alleviate patient suffering.[8] Although the application of narrative medicine can appear widely divergent, its central tasks of attending, representing, and affiliating allow trainees to engage in a rigorous way with narratives.[10]

There is robust evidence that narrative medicine is effective at promoting development of core humanistic skills, including enhancing empathy, improving communication, and strengthening relationships.[8,10,12,14,15,17,19,23] Narrative medicine also benefits observational skills, diagnostic accuracy, and clinical reasoning.[10,18,22,28] A clinician's demonstration of narrative competence has been associated with overall improved patient outcomes, including reduced cancer pain, improved lung function in asthma, and improved immune response following hepatitis B immunization.[24]

Currently, minimal evidence exists on the impact of narrative medicine interventions on academic performance or knowledge retention.[17,20] An application of Vella's principles of adult learning to a narrative andragogy, however, demonstrates how the use of narrative medicine would engage innate learning abilities.[3] The few studies that have examined the impact of narrative medicine on academic performance have shown benefits.[3,17,20] These include long-term improvements in standardized testing as well as overall academic performance following single, time-limited narrative interventions.[17,21]

The aforementioned benefits and the relative flexibility of applying narrative medicine within established educational models provide a strong impetus to consider narrative medicine as a potentially neglected best educational practice. Narrative medicine easily can be incorporated into preclinical and clinical medical training, to help trainees develop a framework for disease models while improving their overall clinical competence. Moreover, narrative training could mitigate diminishment of provider empathy over time and decrease provider burnout.[12,14] When the potential academic gains in tandem with reported improvement in patient outcomes (patient perception of care, pain scores, organ system functioning, and immune health) and provider benefits (improved satisfaction and reduced burnout) are considered, it becomes imperative that the potential of narrative medicine be explored fully.[3,14,17,20,24]

In psychiatry, the benefits of narrative medicine may be even more exaggerated as patients are relied on for full and accurate reports of their internal state and perceptions to formulate and treat. Systematically developing empathy and communication skills through narrative techniques would offer a powerful tool to enhance clinical competence.[8–10,13,14,16,19] Additionally, the potential for narrative medicine to enhance the therapeutic alliance by promoting both patient perceptions and enhanced exploration and mitigation of countertransference could prove a unique and substantive benefit.[13]

Hence, the authors propose a narrative medicine curriculum that could be adapted and applied across a 4-year psychiatry residency (see **Appendices 1–5**). The authors believe this curriculum is flexible and easily could be integrated to individual training program needs. The authors have attempted to leverage what exists within the literature to suggest established techniques with demonstrated efficacy. Additionally, the authors have attempted to design a program that adheres to adult learning principles and builds on itself, optimizing the insights of learning theory. The authors hope that providing such a model may lead to more widespread incorporation of narrative medicine as a potentially underutilized best educational practice.

SUMMARY

This article highlights the importance of narrative medicine in medical education, discusses the potential for narrative medicine within psychiatric residency programs, and proposes an incorporation of narrative medicine in psychiatric postgraduate medical education curricula. The authors approach this recommendation systematically first discussing by the foundational principles of adult learning before introducing the field of narrative medicine and then identifying how the core andragogy within narrative medicine fulfills adult learning principles. Subsequently, narrative medicine's unique benefits within psychiatry are described. Finally, an adaptable 4-year psychiatry residency curriculum to allow for easy adoption and incorporation of these recommendations is proposed.

CLINICS CARE POINTS

- There are 12 principles of adult learning.
- Narrative medicine techniques leverage principles of adult learning.
- Narrative medicine has an established andragogy that is versatile and allows for structured application across many narrative forms.
- The benefits of narrative medicine in promoting empathic connection and exploration of countertransference offer unique benefit to psychiatry.

DISCLOSURE

The authors have nothing to disclose.

REFERENCES

1. Mitchell ML, Courtney M. Improving transfer from the intensive care unit: the development, implementation and evaluation of a brochure based on Knowles' Adult Learning Theory. Int J Nurs Pract 2005;11(6):257–68.
2. Nicklas D, Lane JL, Hanson JL. If You Build It, Will They Come? a hard lesson for enthusiastic medical educators developing a New Curriculum. J Grad Med Educ 2019;11(6):685–90.
3. Vella JK. Learning to listen, learning to teach: the power of dialogue in educating adults. San Francisco: Jossey-Bass; 2002.
4. Smith MK. Malcolm Knowles, informal adult education, self-direction and andragogy. 2002. Available at: https://infed.org/mobi/malcolm-knowles-informal-adult-education-self-direction-and-andragogy/. Accessed May 1, 2020.
5. Blaney PH. Affect and memory: a review. Psychol Bull 1986;99(2):229–46.
6. Fleer M. Affective imagination in science education: determining the emotional nature of scientific and technological learning of young children. Res Sci Educ 2013;43(5):2085–106.
7. Zhu Y, Zhao Y, Ybarra O, et al. Enhanced memory for both threat and neutral information under conditions of intergroup threat. Front Psychol 2015;6:1759.
8. Charon R. The patient-physician relationship. Narrative medicine: a model for empathy, reflection, profession, and trust. JAMA 2001 Oct 17;286(15):1897–902.
9. Charon R, Hermann N, Devlin MJ. Close reading and creative writing in clinical education: teaching attention, representation, and affiliation. Acad Med 2016; 91(3):345–50.
10. Milota MM, van Thiel G, van Delden JJM. Narrative medicine as a medical education tool: A systematic review. Med Teach 2019;41(7):802–10.
11. Huitt W. The information processing approach to cognition. Educational Psychology interactive 2003. Available at: http://www.edpsycinteractive.org/topics/cognition/infoproc.html. Accessed April 27, 2020.
12. Chen PJ, Huang CD, Yeh SJ. Impact of a narrative medicine programme on healthcare providers' empathy scores over time. BMC Med Educ 2017;17(1):108.
13. Deen SR, Mangurian C, Cabaniss DL. Points of contact: using first-person narratives to help foster empathy in psychiatric residents. Acad Psychiatry 2010;34(6): 438–41.
14. Remein CD, Childs E, Pasco JC, et al. Content and outcomes of narrative medicine programmes: a systematic review of the literature through 2019. BMJ Open 2020;10:e031568.

15. Rian J, Hammer R. The practical application of narrative medicine at Mayo Clinic: imagining the scaffold of a worthy house. Cult Med Psychiatry 2013;37(4): 670–80.
16. Muneeb A, Jawaid H, Khalid N, et al. The art of healing through narrative medicine in clinical practice: a reflection. Perm J 2017;21:17–1013.
17. Tsai SL, Ho MJ. Can narrative medicine training improve OSCE performance? Med Educ 2012;46(11):1112–3.
18. Wald HS, Borkan JM, Taylor JS, et al. Fostering and evaluating reflective capacity in medical education: developing the REFLECT rubric for assessing reflective writing. Acad Med 2012;87(1):41–50.
19. Daryazadeh S, Adibi P, Yamani N, et al. Impact of narrative medicine program on improving reflective capacity and empathy of medical students in Iran. J Educ Eval Health Prof 2020;17:3.
20. Weiss T, Swede MJ. Transforming Preprofessional health education through relationship-centered care and narrative medicine. Teach Learn Med 2019; 31(2):222–33.
21. Yang N, Xiao H, Cao Y, et al. Does narrative medicine education improve nursing students' empathic abilities and academic achievement? A randomised controlled trial. J Int Med Res 2018;46(8):3306–17.
22. Liao HC, Wang YH. Storytelling in medical education: narrative medicine as a resource for interdisciplinary collaboration. Int J Environ Res Public Health 2020;17(4):1135.
23. Barber S, Moreno-Leguizamon CJ. Can narrative medicine e'ducation contribute to the delivery of compassionate care? A review of the literature. Med Humanit 2017;43(3):199–203.
24. Zaharias G. What is narrative-based medicine? Narrative-based medicine 1. Can Fam Physician 2018;64(3):176–80.
25. Cutler JL, Harding KJ, Mozian SA, et al. Discrediting the notion "working with 'crazies' will make you 'crazy'": addressing stigma and enhancing empathy in medical student education. Adv Health Sci Educ Theor Pract 2009;14(4): 487–502.
26. Bromley E, Braslow JT. Teaching critical thinking in psychiatric training: a role for the social sciences. Am J Psychiatry 2008;165(11):1396–401.
27. Garrison D, Lyness JM, Frank JB, et al. Qualitative analysis of medical student impressions of a narrative exercise in the third-year psychiatry clerkship. Acad Med 2011;86(1):85–9.
28. Maurer MS, Costley AW, Miller PA, et al. The Columbia Cooperative Aging Program: an interdisciplinary and interdepartmental approach to geriatric education for medical interns. J Am Geriatr Soc 2006;54(3):520–6.
29. Seligman MEP, Csikszentmihalyi M. Positive psychology: an introduction. Am Psychol 2000;55(1):5–14.
30. White M, Richards G. Psychiatrists' dress and address. Br J Psychiatry 1998; 172:95.
31. Schildkrout B. Am I looking at a malignant melanoma? New York Times; 2008. Available at: nytimes.com.
32. Savodnik I. Psychiatry's sick compulsion: turning weaknesses into diseases. Los Angeles Times; 2006. Available at: latimes.com.
33. Grob GN. Origins of DSM-I: a study in appearance and reality. Am J Psychiatry 1991;148(4):421–31.
34. Carlson GA, Glovinsky I. The concept of bipolar disorder in children: a history of the bipolar controversy. Child Adolesc Psychiatr Clin N Am 2009;18(2):257–71, vii.

35. Goldney RD. From mania and melancholia to the bipolar disorders spectrum: a brief history of controversy. Aust N Z J Psychiatry 2012;46(4):306–12.
36. Healy D. Shaping the intimate: influences on the experience of everyday nerves. Soc Stud Sci 2004;34(2):219–45.
37. Sass LA. Madness and modernism: insanity in the light of modern art, literature, and thought. Oxford University Press; Revised edition; 2017.
38. Obeyesekere G. "Depression and the Work of Culture". In: Kleinman A, editor. Culture and depression: studies in the anthropology and cross-cultural psychiatry of affect and disorder. Berkeley. CA: Univ. of California Pr; 1985.
39. Scheper-Hughes N. 'Mental' in 'Southie': individual, family, and community responses to psychosis in South Boston. Cult Med Psychiatry 1987;11(1):53–78.
40. Braslow JT, University of California P. Mental ills and bodily cures: psychiatric treatment in the first half of the twentieth century. Berkeley (CA): University of California Press; 1997.
41. Braslow JT. History and evidence-based medicine: lessons from the history of somatic treatments from the 1900s to the 1950s. Ment Health Serv Res 1999;1(4):231–40.
42. Braslow JT, Duan N, Starks SL, et al. Generalizability of studies on mental health treatment and outcomes, 1981 to 1996. Psychiatr Serv 2005;56(10):1261–8.
43. Bromley E. Stimulating a normal adjustment: misbehavior, amphetamines, and the electroencephalogram at the Bradley Home for children. J Hist Behav Sci 2006;42(4):379–98.
44. Karlinsky H. The Horse Boy—attending to the stories our patients tell us. Acad Psychiatry 2013;37(4):271–5.
45. Edwards-Leeper L, Spack NP. Psychological evaluation and medical treatment of transgender youth In an interdisciplinary "Gender Management Service" (GeMS) in a Major Pediatric Center. J Homosex 2012;59(3):321–36.
46. Watkins CE Jr, Hook JN, Owen J, et al. Multicultural Orientation in Psychotherapy Supervision: Cultural Humility, Cultural Comfort, and Cultural Opportunities. Am J Psychother 2019;72(2):38–46, https://doi.org/10.1176/appi.psychothe.
47. Lakoff A. The anxieties of globalization: antidepressant sales and economic crisis in Argentina. Soc Stud Sci 2004;34(2):247–69.
48. Solomon A. The noonday demon: an atlas of depression. New York, NY: Scribner: Simon & Schuster; 2002.
49. Saks ER. The center cannot hold: my journey through madness. New York: Hyperion; 2007.
50. Estroff SE. Making it crazy: an ethnography of psychiatric clients in an american community. Berkeley, CA: Univ. of California Press; 1981.
51. Edgerton RB. The cloak of competence: stigma in the lives of the mentally retarded. Berkeley, CA: University of California Press; 1967.
52. Rhodes LA. Emptying beds: the work of an emergency psychiatric unit. Berkeley, CA: University of California Press; 1991.
53. Allan C. Summerscapes: a midsummer day's nightmare. New York Times; 2006.
54. Robbins ML, Wright RC, María López A, et al. Interpersonal positive reframing in the daily lives of couples coping with breast cancer. J Psychosoc Oncol 2019; 37(2):160–77.
55. Graham K, Patterson T, Justice T, et al. "It's Not a Great Boulder, It's Just a Piece of Baggage": Older Women's reflections on healing from childhood sexual abuse. J Interpers Violence 2020. 886260520916270.
56. Ridgway P. ReStorying psychiatric disability: learning from first person recovery narratives. Psychiatr Rehabil J 2001;24(4):335–43.

APPENDIX: PROPOSED CURRICULUM

Appendix 1
Introduction to narrative techniques course

Session	Central Questions	Narratives
1	What is narrative medicine?	Charon R. The patient-physician relationship. Narrative medicine: a model for empathy, reflection, profession, and trust. *JAMA*. 2001;286(15):1897–1902 https://doi.org/10.1001/jama.286.15.1897[8]
2	Why narrative medicine?	Remein CDiF, Childs E,Pasco JC, et al. Content and outcomes of narrative medicine programmes: a systematic review of the literature through 2019. BMJ Open 2020;10:e031568 https://doi.org/10.1136/bmjopen-2019-031568[14] Milota, M.M.; van Thiel, G.T.M.W.; van Delden, J.J.M. Narrative medicine as a medical education tool: A systematic review. Med. Teach. 2019, 41, 802–810[10]

Appendix 2
Becoming a psychiatrist

Session	Central Questions	Narratives	Homework
1	What did friends and family say when you told them you were going into psychiatry?		Find a fictional representation of a psychiatrist in literature or the media that you can identify with and bring to share.
2	What is a psychiatrist?	Seligman ME, Csikszentmihalyi M. Positive psychology. An introduction. *Am Psychol*. 2000;55(1):5-14. https://doi.org/10.1037//0003-066x.55.1.5[29] M. White, G. Richards. "Psychiatrists' dress and address." Br J Psychiatry. 172:95. 1998[30]	Describe an attending who embodies your idea of a psychiatrist; write a 1-page imagined or actual encounter from your own, the patient's, or the attending's perspective.
3	What does one lose in becoming a psychiatrist, and what does one gain?	Schildkrout, B. Am I looking at a malignant melanoma? *The New York Times*, New York, NY: 2008[31]	Close reading of *Los Angeles Times* article "Psychiatry's sick compulsion: turning weaknesses into diseases"[32]
4	What do you say to respond to critics of psychiatry or those who idealize it?	Savodnik, I. Psychiatry's sick compulsion: turning weaknesses into diseases. *Los Angeles Times*. Los Angeles: 2006[32]	N/A

Appendix 3 Psychiatric diagnosis			
Session	Central Task/Question	Narratives	Homework
1	Review of the history of psychiatric diagnosis	*Diagnostic and Statistical Manual of Mental Disorders* (prior and current versions) Grob. "Origins of DSM-I: a study in appearance and reality." Am J Psychiatry148(4). 1991[33]	Choose 1 of the narratives for the next session and write a reflection piece.
2	How do we apply labels?	Carlson GA, Glovinsky I. The concept of bipolar disorder in children: a history of the bipolar controversy. *Child Adolesc Psychiatr Clin N Am.* 2009;18(2):257-vii https://doi.org/10.1016/j.chc.2008.11.003[34] Goldney RD. From mania and melancholia to the bipolar disorders spectrum: a brief history of controversy. *Aust N Z J Psychiatry.* 2012;46(4):306-312 https://doi.org/10.1177/0004867412440195[35]	Identify another controversial diagnosis and write a piece where you imagine yourself having to evaluate a patient presenting with that diagnosis.
3	Where does normal end and pathology begin?	Healy D. Shaping the intimate: influences on the experience of everyday nerves. *Soc Stud Sci.* 2004;34(2):219-245 https://doi.org/10.1177/0306312704042620[36] Sass, LA. Madness and modernism: insanity in the light of modern art, literature, and thought. Oxford University Press; Revised edition; 2017[37]	Identify a poem— write an imagined mental status examination of the author.
4	How does culture influence psychiatric diagnosis?	G. Obeyesekere. "Depression and the Work of Culture." In Kleinman A, editor. Culture and depression: studies in the anthropology and cross-cultural psychiatry of affect and disorder. Berkeley, CA: Univ. of California Pr; 1985[38] Scheper-Hughes N. 'Mental' in 'Southie': individual, family, and community responses to psychosis in South Boston Culture, Medicine & Psychiatry. 1987; 11(1):53–78[39]	N/A

Appendix 4			
Psychiatric treatment			
Session	Central Topics	Narratives	Homework
1	Where did we begin?	Braslow, JT. Mental ills and bodily cures: psychiatric treatment in the first half of the twentieth century. Berkeley: University of California Press; 1997[40]	Write the story of the first patient you treated—how did you choose a treatment? What evidence did you use?
2	Evidence-based medicine	Braslow JT. History and evidence-based medicine: lessons from the history of somatic treatments from the 1900s to the 1950s. Ment Health Serv Res. 1999; 1(4):231–40[41]	Identify the top 5 clinical trials that guide clinician practice—ask mentors/ supervisors which trials influenced them.
3	Clinical trials: the good, the bad, and the ugly	Braslow JT, Duan N, Starks SL, Polo A, Bromley E, Wells KB. Generalizability of studies on mental health treatment and outcomes, 1981–1996. Psychiatr Serv. 2005; 56(10):1261–8 [PubMed: 16215192][42]	What makes a patient vulnerable? Are some populations more vulnerable? Why? Write a paragraph from the perspective of a vulnerable patient from the waiting room at a first visit.
4	Vulnerable populations— children, prisoners	Bromley E. Stimulating a normal adjustment: Misbehavior, amphetamines, and the electroencephalogram at the Bradley Home for children. J Hist Behav Sci. 2006; 42(4):379–398 [PubMed: 17024684][43] Karlinsky H. The Horse Boy— attending to the stories our patients tell us. *Acad Psychiatry.* 2013; 37(4):271-275. https://doi.org/ 10.1176/appi.ap.13040048[44]	Describe the spectrum of gender and sexual identities.

(continued on next page)

Appendix 4 (continued)			
Session	Central Topics	Narratives	Homework
5	Gender and sexuality: What is in a word?	Laura Edwards-Leeper PhD & Norman P. Spack MD (2012) Psychological evaluation and medical treatment of transgender youth in an interdisciplinary "Gender Management Service" (GeMS) in a major pediatric center, Journal of Homosexuality, 59:3, 321–336, https://doi.org/10.1080/00918369.2012.653302[45]	Read Watkins CE Jr, Hook JN, Owen J, DeBlaere C, Davis DE, Van Tongeren DR. Multicultural Orientation in Psychotherapy Supervision: Cultural Humility, Cultural Comfort, and Cultural Opportunities. Am J Psychother. 2019;72(2):38-46 https://doi.org/10.1176/appi.psychotherapy.20180040.[46] Consider 1 patient encounter in which you either used a position of cultural humility or did not, and how such a frame has an impact on the work.
6	Cultural humility: the unknown unknowns	Watkins CE Jr, Hook JN, Owen J, DeBlaere C, Davis DE, Van Tongeren DR. Multicultural orientation in psychotherapy supervision: cultural humility, cultural comfort, and cultural opportunities. Am J Psychother. 2019;72(2):38-46 https://doi.org/10.1176/appi.psychotherapy.20180040[46]	Find a current drug advertisement, and imagine you are a patient with that disorder; write a piece exploring what it is like to watch that advertisement.
7	Marketing and medication	Lakoff A. The anxieties of globalization: antidepressant sales and economic crisis in Argentina. *Soc Stud Sci.* 2004;34(2):247-269. https://doi.org/10.1177/0306312704042624[47]	N/A

Appendix 5
Illness experience

Session	Central Topics	Narratives	Homework
1	Depression	Solomon, A. The noonday demon: An atlas of depression. New York: Scribner; 2002[48]	Choose either a first-person narrative or artwork: https://academic.oup.com/ schizophreniabulletin/ pages/first_person_accounts *or view the patient artwork; reflect on your internal experience. Saks, ER. The center cannot hold: My journey through madness. New York: Hyperion; 2007[49]
2	Psychosis	https://academic.oup. com/schizophreniabulletin/ pages/first_person_accounts Cahalan, S. Brain on fire: My month of madness. New York: Simon and Schuster; 2012 Saks, ER. The center cannot hold: My journey through madness. New York: Hyperion; 2007[49]	Steinbeck, John. Of Mice and Men. New York: Penguin Books; 1994 Read a self-selected 5-page excerpt from *Of Mice and Men* and prepare to discuss in class.
3	Intellectual disability	Estroff, SE. Making it crazy: an ethnography of psychiatric clients in an American community. Berkeley: University of California Press; 1981[50] Edgerton, RB. The cloak of competence: Stigma in the lives of the mentally retarded. Berkeley: University of California Press; 1967[51]	Do staff make assumptions about patient's lives? Are they correct? What function do these assumptions serve?
4	Institutio-nalization	Rhodes, LA. Emptying beds: The work of an emergency psychiatric unit. Berkeley: University of California Press; 1991[52] Allan, C. Summerscapes: A midsummer day's nightmare. *The New York Times*. New York, NY: 2006.[53]	Imagine a recent irritating though not extremely distressing experience. Try to shift your experience to view the "silver lining". Did any good come out of the experience? Why did it happen?

(continued on next page)

Appendix 5 (*continued*)			
Session	Central Topics	Narratives	Homework
5	Meaning-making	Robbins ML, Wright RC, María López A, Weihs K. Interpersonal positive reframing in the daily lives of couples coping with breast cancer. *J Psychosoc Oncol.* 2019;37(2):160-177 https://doi.org/10.1080/07347332.2018.1555198[54] Graham K, Patterson T, Justice T, Rapsey C. "It's not a great boulder, it's just a piece of baggage": Older women's reflections on healing from childhood sexual abuse [published online ahead of print, 2020 Apr 20]. *J Interpers Violence.* 2020;886260520916270 https://doi.org/10.1177/0886260520916270[55]	Find a story of someone who has experienced something difficult (real or fictional); how do they talk about it? How does this influence how they experience the world?
6	Recovery	Ridgway, P. (2001). ReStorying psychiatric disability: Learning from first person recovery narratives. Psychiatric Rehabilitation Journal, 24(4), 335–343. https://doi.org/10.1037/h0095071[56]	

Fostering Careers in Medical Education

Adrienne T. Gerken, MD[a],[*],[1], David L. Beckmann, MD, MPH[b],[1],
Theodore A. Stern, MD[c]

KEYWORDS

- Education • Medical education • Careers • Psychiatry • Academic psychiatry
- Clinician educator • Diversity

KEY POINTS

- Early exposure to information about career trajectories in medical education, as well as mentorship in developing an identity as a medical educator, is important in creating and maintaining excellence in psychiatric education.
- Mentorship, protected time for educational research and teaching, exposure to academic career paths, and an understanding of the promotion process are all factors that facilitate academic careers.
- Psychiatry residents should develop a core set of teaching skills, with more advanced skills training available for residents with a specific interest in medical education.
- Training programs should strongly consider the creation of clinician-educator programs or tracks, while departments should create clear promotion pathways for clinician-educators.
- Departments and training programs should seek to diversify their faculty and residency programs and to support those who identify as underrepresented in medicine and gender-diverse individuals, while simultaneously undertaking self-examination and steps to create a positive and inclusive environment.

BACKGROUND

From its earliest days, the apprenticeship model of medical education has relied on the willingness and aptitude of physicians to teach their craft. Fortunately, medical education has progressed substantially since the days when residents were charged to "see one, do one, teach one" and sent on their way. As they progress in their own

[a] McLean Hospital Psychiatry Residency Program, Harvard Medical School, Massachusetts General Hospital, McLean Hospital, Mailstop 229, Belmont, MA 02478, USA; [b] McLean Hospital Psychiatry Residency Program, Harvard Medical School, Massachusetts General Hospital, 15 Parkman Street, WACC 812, Boston, MA 02114, USA; [c] Avery D. Weisman Psychiatry Consultation Service, Harvard Medical School, Thomas P. Hackett Center for Scholarship in Psychosomatic Medicine, Office for Clinical Careers, Massachusetts General Hospital, 55 Fruit Street, Warren 606, Boston, MA 02114, USA
[1] Co-first authors.
* Corresponding author.
E-mail address: agerken@partners.org

Psychiatr Clin N Am 44 (2021) 283–294
https://doi.org/10.1016/j.psc.2020.12.007
0193-953X/21/© 2021 Elsevier Inc. All rights reserved.

education, today's psychiatry residents can learn *about* teaching and choose from a diverse array of career paths that require, and value, teaching skills.

A core set of teaching skills is essential to the practice of psychiatry and residents should not graduate without these skills, regardless of their planned practice setting. The Accreditation Council for Graduate Medical Education (ACGME) Psychiatry Milestones include a specific milestone dedicated to teaching,[1] with target skills for graduation that include the ability to deliver formal didactic presentations and the ability to use feedback on teaching effectively.

Within academic practice, many careers are available to psychiatrist-educators; residents should learn about these pathways early enough in training to pursue advanced opportunities during residency. In addition, many psychiatry residency programs have created clinician educator programs (CEPs) or clinician educator tracks (CETs) that offer organized opportunities to explore advanced concepts, practice teaching skills, pursue scholarship, and be mentored in medical education.

A robust, diverse, and appropriately compensated faculty of clinician-educators is a prerequisite for assisting residents in the pursuit of medical education careers. Protected time for teaching and mentorship allows clinician-educator faculty to hone their teaching skills, deliver high-quality didactics, mentor residents interested in careers as educators, and create scholarly works that include resident mentees. Furthermore, residents are more likely to embark on careers in medical education when they see that their institutions value clinician-educators, both financially and academically.

DISCUSSION
Career Paths in Medical Education

Exposing residents to information about career opportunities in medical education increases their awareness of the myriad options available, and assists them in their development as educators.[2] Medical students identify mentorship, protected time for research and teaching, exposure to academic career trajectories, and an understanding of the promotion process as factors that facilitate academic careers.[3]

Academic promotions

Paths to promotion and tenure vary by institution, and promotion criteria are often so byzantine that even long-term faculty members struggle to comprehend them. However, it is a disservice to residents if they are not exposed to the principles of promotion so that those who choose an academic career can make informed decisions as they seek employment.

For programs affiliated with universities and/or medical schools, it may be most useful to teach general principles of promotion while using the program's academic institution as an example, because many residents stay (at least initially) where they trained. For community-based programs, general principles should be covered; it may also be useful to discuss ways in which community psychiatrists can be involved in university-based academic psychiatry.

Residents who are considering an academic career should understand the difference between tenure and nontenure tracks and the benefits and drawbacks of each path. Specific promotion paths (or areas of excellence) should be explained and the criteria for promotion should be shared with residents. Residents should receive mentorship from faculty having different career trajectories, who can speak about their choices and how those choices influenced their lives (and work-life balance).

Education-related tracks are relatively new compared with clinical expertise and investigation tracks.[4] In general, promotion of educators focuses on educational scholarship and/or leadership.[5] Education-related paths to promotion are often less well-defined, or not up-to-date on newer educational formats, including use of social media.[6]

Residents should understand that some institutions have an "up or out" policy (a "tenure clock") with those not promoted moving to the nontenure track. This structure tends to place a lower value on nontenure positions. However, residents should appreciate that the choice to pursue a tenure versus nontenure track should be based on their goals and values, not on presumed prestige. Similarly, they should understand that fulfilling and valued teaching positions exist outside of traditional academic settings.

Any discussion of academic promotions is incomplete without acknowledging historical and present-day inequities in the process. Women, gender-diverse individuals (eg, those who are transgender or gender-nonconforming) and people of color have long been passed over in the promotions process.[7,8] Residents should be educated about overt and implicit bias in academia and graduating residents should be connected with mentors who can help them navigate the process.

Career paths in psychiatric education

To encourage and support potential clinician-educators, trainees (such as psychiatry residents) must understand the range of careers in medical education (**Table 1**). The nature of these roles varies dramatically between medical centers and departments. However, most academic medical centers, particularly those with larger psychiatry departments, have many or most of these positions, which we describe as follows.

First, not all academic departments are willing, or have the required resources, to support dedicating a significant portion of a clinician's time to teaching. Instead,

Table 1
Educator roles: undergraduate medical education, graduate medical education, and hospital-based

Medical School/Undergraduate Medical Education	Residency/Graduate Medical Education	Hospital-Based/Other
Vice Chair of Education	Program Director	Chief Academic Officer/ GME Office Director
Deans of: • Education • Students/Student Affairs • Diversity • Wellness • Faculty Development	Associate Program Director(s)	Medical Director/Clinical Director
Director of Medical Student Education	Assistant Program Director(s)	Clinical supervisor (physician assistant or nurse practitioner)
Clerkship Director	Special Programs Directors: • Clinician-Educator Program/Track • Psychotherapy • Research	Interprofessional teammate
Clinical preceptor	Didactic course leaders	Education to the general public
Interprofessional schools (eg, didactics for physician assistant or nurse practitioner students)	Teaching attendings, supervisors, mentors	

models include clinical-teacher roles (eg, an inpatient attending on a teaching unit with a smaller patient panel but expectations to educate the residents they work with) and leadership roles with significant administrative responsibilities, such as curriculum design and oversight of learners (eg, residency Program Directors or directors of undergraduate psychiatry clerkships). The nature of these roles should be clarified, and instruction and mentorship should be provided in both the mechanics of teaching and performance of administrative work.

Therefore, careers in medical education can be divided into psychiatrists who focus on undergraduate medical education (UME), graduate medical education (GME), and other learners (eg, faculty, staff in other specialties or allied health professionals, and members of the general public).

At most university-based programs, medical students far outnumber psychiatry trainees. Medical students are a diverse group in terms of their experience, strengths, and interests (including their level of interest in psychiatry). Therefore, working with medical students can be both rewarding and challenging.

Psychiatrists also have an important role in the preclinical portion of medical school as well as working with students on the wards in their core psychiatry rotations and advanced electives. Some schools have a dedicated administrator to oversee preclinical instruction in psychiatry; most medical schools also have an identified clerkship director whose job includes designing, evaluating, and overseeing the core clinical psychiatry experiences. Some psychiatry departments may have a faculty member who oversees learners across all levels of UME in the specialty (preclinical, core clinical, advanced elective). In addition, medical schools have higher administrative positions for medical educators, notably a Dean of Students, who oversees medical education for all medical students. Although most medical schools have only one such position, the interpersonal focus of psychiatric training may be advantageous for psychiatrists interested in this role.

Equivalent or analogous roles exist in GME. Many academic medical centers have ample opportunity for psychiatrists to provide clinical teaching on rotations, during formal didactics, and during clinical supervision. These roles might be required of faculty and might be compensated. Residency programs often have clinician-educators oversee subsets of the educational experiences, such as a resident's time on inpatient or outpatient settings.

ACGME rules require residency training program to be overseen by a Program Director (a board-certified psychiatrist with at least 3 years of educational or administrative experience who must continue to engage in clinical practice).[9] Many larger programs have additional program leadership roles, including one or more associate and/or assistant program director(s). These roles may be appropriate for junior faculty, as they provide a learning experience for educators interested in becoming a program director or having another role in medical education leadership. Some larger departments have a role that oversees psychiatric training at all levels, such as a vice chair for education.

As in UME, higher-level hospital administrative roles may draw from all specialties, and interested psychiatrists may consider such positions. Most academic medical centers have an internal office of GME, often led by a chief academic officer. Although such offices have traditionally drawn heavily from Internal Medicine, diverse perspectives are beneficial in creating hospital-wide educational policies.

Finally, roles exist outside of academic systems that offer opportunities for interested clinician-educators. In fact, as psychiatric care increasingly falls to primary care providers and midlevel psychiatric professionals (nurse practitioners and physician assistants), the need for experienced and skilled psychiatrist supervisors has been increasing. Many academic, community, and private groups employ psychiatrists to provide consultation and supervision to practitioners who have completed their training, but whose training has a different focus or is not as robust as that offered in psychiatric residency training programs. Supervision, formal interprofessional education (such as being the medical director of an interprofessional group), and even education of the general public (via writing for the lay press, giving media interviews, consulting to schools or community groups) are all roles outside of the traditional academic ranks that benefit from strong knowledge base in educational principles. Programs should ensure that trainees are aware of these diverse opportunities in medical education. Formal avenues (through mentorship or didactics) have increased awareness of, and interest in, these paths.[2]

Teaching Skills

All graduates of psychiatric residency programs should have accrued a core set of teaching skills (**Table 2**). These skills are broadly applicable, whether a resident intends to become a clinical teacher on an inpatient unit or to skillfully educate their patients in a private practice. Residents with a strong interest in medical education benefit from having a more advanced set of skills, which they can begin to develop in residency (see **Table 2**).

Essential teaching skills

All residents should graduate with the ability to teach a variety of group sizes (one-on-one, small group, larger group, and lectures) across a variety of settings (including in-person and online). They should have experience with informal teaching (such as bedside teaching or brief "chalk talks") and more formal teaching (such as conferences).

Residents should develop a basic understanding about how to plan a didactic or talk, regardless of its length or setting, and should have practice in planning teaching

Table 2 Essential and advanced teaching skills for residents	
Core Resident Teaching Skills	**Advanced Resident Teaching Skills**
Basic content and skills: • Adult learning theory • Clinical teaching • Delivering feedback • Supervision (trainees, other physicians, multidisciplinary staff) • Delivery of talks and seminars Opportunities: • Rotation-based and clinical teaching • Morbidity and mortality conferences, departmental conferences	Advanced content and skills: • Administrative skills for clinician-educators • How to mentor • Advanced teaching techniques (eg, flipped classroom) • Technology in teaching • Teaching for various group sizes and venues • Curriculum design • Models of evaluation and promotion (eg, milestones or entrustable professional activities) Opportunities: • Mentorship by teaching faculty • Education-related committee membership • Resident fellowship nominations (eg, Association for Academic Psychiatry) • Professional memberships • National meetings • Grand Rounds • Academic scholarship

sessions.[10] In addition to rotation-related teaching opportunities, programs may offer residents the chance to present at morbidity and mortality conferences or other departmental conferences. Designating a specific faculty member or mentor to help residents prepare these presentations is key to helping them feel supported in "high-visibility" teaching settings.

Most importantly, residents should have ample opportunity to teach and receive feedback on their teaching throughout residency. Feedback should be formative rather than summative, and should focus on the residents' teaching goals.[11]

Ideally, residents will receive feedback from peers as well as from supervisors. Peer feedback can be incredibly effective and is often perceived as less threatening than feedback from supervisors. The Peer Observation of Teaching model can be used as a framework for feedback, while also teaching residents how to deliver effective feedback.[12]

In addition to learning how to deliver content-driven teaching sessions, residents should learn specific content and skills related to education. All residents should be familiar with the principles of adult learning, including strategies for incorporating adult learning theory into their own talks.[13] They should learn how to deliver high-quality, actionable, feedback to supervisees (medical students, more junior residents, and multidisciplinary staff) and peers.[14] In addition, they should learn how to use vulnerability in teaching to connect with trainees and create a "safe space" for the learner.[15]

Advanced teaching skills

Residents who are interested in teaching or who intend to choose a career in education should have access to additional content and opportunities. Some programs offer these through electives or a dedicated CEP or CET. In programs in which these resources are not available, residents may pursue education-related courses through their hospitals, medical schools, or professional organizations (such as the Association for Academic Psychiatry [AAP]). Residents with a strong interest in medical education benefit from mentorship around teaching, pursuing educational careers, and academic scholarship.

Residents who pursue advanced teaching skills should understand and practice techniques for curriculum design.[16] They benefit from experience with advanced teaching techniques, including problem-based learning,[17,18] team-based learning,[19] simulation,[20] just-in-time teaching,[21] and flipped-classroom approaches.[22]

Education-oriented residents should have familiarity with, and practice using, technology in teaching.[23] These technologies may include audience response systems,[24] app-based learning, online discussion boards, online cases and/or instructional videos and tutorials,[25] adaptive learning technology,[26] and use (and even creation of) podcasts.[27]

In addition to learning about learner assessment,[28] they should learn the pros and cons of various models of evaluation and promotion, such as the Milestones[29] and Entrustable Professional Activities.[30] They should begin to build a skillset to help learners who are struggling to meet benchmarks.[31]

Interested residents may even begin to learn the "meta skills" of educational administration, often learned through chief resident positions. These skills include how to foster positive culture in organizations and learning environments.[32] They may begin to serve as a formal mentor to more junior residents, particularly in a chief resident role.

On an institutional level, trainees also benefit from opportunities for membership on education-related committees (such as the residency's Educational Policy Committee) and opportunities to present (or co-present) at departmental meetings, such as Grand Rounds. Outside their home institution, they benefit from support for membership in professional organizations dedicated to teaching, funding for national meetings, and nomination to education-related fellowships (such as those offered by the AAP and Association of American Medical Colleges).

Educational scholarship
Residents interested in careers in medical education benefit from beginning to build their "educator portfolio," including educational scholarship. The term "educational scholarship" goes well beyond educational research or published articles and includes creation of teaching materials, development of assessment methods, publication of curricula (for example, via MedEdPORTAL), creation of Web-based tools or videos, writing educational apps, and more.

Mentorship is key to success in academic scholarship, and educational scholarship is no exception. Residents should receive assistance in building a network of mentors, including at least one mentor whose focus is on medical education. Additional mentorship around specific content areas or educational research may be beneficial, depending on the resident's goals.

Clinician-Educator Programs and Tracks

Specialized training for residents interested in medical education can take many forms. At the most basic level, programs may offer elective time that can be used for medical education electives, either predefined or arranged by the resident.

Longitudinal experiences in medical education can be organized as clinician-educator programs or tracks (CEPs or CETs, respectively). These can be organized as a separate National Resident Matching Program track into which residents match[33] or as an elective that residents join after matching. The latter type can be limited to a certain number of residents or include all residents who are interested and meet the application requirements. The program may be housed within psychiatry or offered across multiple residency disciplines.[34] The didactic content may be delivered during the regular resident workday or as a separate series of after-work didactics. There are advantages and disadvantages to each model, so decisions about how to shape the track will depend on the structure of the program and the needs of the residents.

Regardless of structure, CEPs or CETs are likely to include didactic content or workshops, individual or group mentorship, teaching opportunities (with observation and feedback), and scholarly activity.[33,34]

CEPs or CETs are excellent investments in workforce development. Residents who receive specific mentorship around their academic goals are more likely to pursue an academic trajectory,[3,35] enabling them with teaching skills; this will provide a natural pool of future faculty with specific skills in medical education.

Finally, it is worth noting that there a number of journals dedicated to or prominently feature articles about medical education (and in some cases, specifically psychiatry education). MedEdPORTAL is a peer-reviewed online-only journal specifically for publishing work related to this topic, and several online and paper journals are also very good resources for anyone interested in the topic (**Box 1**). Whether through a CEP or CET or through other avenues, trainees who are particularly interested in medical education career should be encouraged to look to these resources for up-to-date information and guidance.

Diversity in Psychiatric Education

A future that is brighter and more just requires special attention to promoting careers in academic medicine for people from ethnic and racial minority groups. Physicians who identify as underrepresented in medicine (URM; namely those who are Black or

African American, Latinx or Hispanic, and Native American, Alaskan, Hawaiian, or other Pacific Islander) made up only 8% of faculty in academic medicine in 2015,[36] despite comprising nearly one-third of the US population.[37] While we focus here on racial and ethnic minorities (who are more likely to be affected by multigenerational structural barriers), similar disparities exist (although are less well characterized) for other minority groups, particularly gender-diverse individuals.[38] In a profession historically dominated by white men, women remain underrepresented as well, particularly in the higher-ranking positions. A 2018 survey found that women comprised 42% of the workforce in academic psychiatry; this included only 25% of full professors and only 9% of departmental chairs.[39]

A variety of structural factors, including disproportionate levels of poverty and lower levels of access to high-quality education, role models, and mentors, results in fewer URM persons joining the ranks of medical faculty in the first place. Structural factors continue to impact the careers of URM physicians who do become faculty and academic medical centers must take steps to address these issues. URM faculty members publish fewer than two-thirds as many papers as their white counterparts and are about half as likely to be promoted to professor or to stay in academic medicine.[8] URM faculty have ambitious career aspirations but are less likely to perceive a culture of inclusivity and equity compared with their non-URM counterparts.[40]

In psychiatry, Black and Latinx physicians made up only 3.8% and 3.6% of faculty, respectively, in 2018.[41] These numbers fall further when looking at more advanced academic ranks; full professors are particularly underrepresented by Black (1.7%) and Latinx (2.5%) physicians. These numbers represent only a very small increase from a decade ago, less even than the proportional increase of these racial and ethnic groups nationally.[41]

The many reasons that URMs are less likely to join and remain at academic medical centers are myriad, and beyond the scope of this discussion. To create diverse departments, it is incumbent on medical centers and departments to address disparities,

---

Box 1
Medical and psychiatric education journals

Academic Medicine

Academic Psychiatry

Advances in Health Sciences Education

BMC Medical Education

The Clinical Teacher

Evaluation in the Health Professions

Journal of the American Medical Association

Journal of Continuing Education in the Health Professions

Journal of Graduate Medical Education

MedEdPORTAL (online only)

Medical Education

Medical Science Educator

Medical Teacher

Teaching and Learning in Medicine

including structural and cultural biases, overt discrimination from colleagues and patients, and lack of role models and mentors.

Much has been written about the benefits of a diverse faculty for all learners, and downstream, for patient care.[42] We emphasize that a lack of diversity tends to be self-perpetuating; that a racially homogeneous faculty decreases the availability of URM mentors and role models and runs counter to a culture of inclusivity. If academic medical centers and psychiatry departments value structurally competent care of diverse patient populations, a diverse workforce is paramount. Ensuring this diversity among matriculants and graduates requires prioritizing diversity among faculty and among physicians in leadership positions. Therefore, organizations must examine what steps they are taking to ensure that diverse candidates, with respect to factors such as gender, sexual identity, religion, and particularly URM status, are provided with the necessary mentorship, resources, and academic culture to foster and promote careers in medical education.

SUMMARY

Academic medical centers are increasingly recognizing the importance of emphasizing the skillset of clinician-educators in formal medical education, although avenues for support, mentorship, and promotion still lag behind most institutions' emphasis on the teaching and supporting of clinical-related and research-related skills. To allow individuals (including psychiatry trainees) to excel in academic medicine, and particularly to pursue a career as a clinician-educator, medical centers must provide learners with the necessary skills, knowledge, and opportunities. This includes educating all psychiatry residents in basic teaching skills, and ideally providing interested learners additional instruction through advanced electives, a clinician educator track or program, and formal mentorship from senior faculty working in medical education. In addition to concrete teaching skills, these opportunities and relationships provide trainees with an understanding of what opportunities exist in medical education and create pathways for residents to pursue. Programs should provide information about a variety of education-related careers and opportunities, including those in UME, GME, and less traditional teaching roles (such as interprofessional supervision or educating the public). Particular attention should be paid to providing mentorship and other education resources to URM trainees, as a diverse workforce in medical education is necessary to promote a stronger and more inclusive workforce for future generations of physicians.

CLINICS CARE POINTS

- Most academic psychiatrists have traditionally pursued promotion either through a pathway related to clinical excellence and innovation, or a pathway related to research and investigation. We recommend that psychiatry departments in academic medical centers consider joining a growing trend of departments offering a third promotional track: that of the clinician educator.

- For clinical education to continuously improve, emphasis on developing an identity as an educator should begin while psychiatrists are still in training.

- Psychiatry training programs would offer multiple avenues for learning about careers in clinical education, as well as the knowledge and skills required to excel in this path.

- Robust instruction in clinical education may include teaching seminars and/or clinical rotations geared toward all residents, advanced teaching electives for particularly interested trainees, and/or a CET or CEP.

- Although a career in medical education may feel daunting for all learners, there are additional structural barriers for trainees from groups who are URM. Particular care must be taken to provide mentorship and an educational culture that acts to overcome these barriers.

DISCLOSURE

The authors have nothing to disclose.

REFERENCES

1. Reporting M. The psychiatry milestone project. J Graduate Med Educ 2014; 6:285.
2. Fernandez CR, Lucas R, Soto-Greene M, et al. Introducing trainees to academic medicine career roles and responsibilities. MedEdPORTAL 2017;13:10653.
3. Sánchez J, Peters L, Lee-Rey E, et al. Racial and ethnic minority medical students' perceptions of and interest in careers in academic medicine. Acad Med 2013;88(9):1299–307.
4. Register SJ, King KM. Promotion and tenure: Application of scholarship of teaching and learning, and scholarship of engagement criteria to health professions education. Health Professions Education 2018;4(1):39–47.
5. Atasoylu AA, Wright SM, Beasley BW, et al. Promotion criteria for clinician-educators. J Gen Intern Med 2003;18(9):711–6.
6. Ryan MS, Tucker C, DiazGranados D, et al. How are clinician-educators evaluated for educational excellence? A survey of promotion and tenure committee members in the United States. Med Teach 2019;41(8):927–33.
7. Carr PL, Gunn C, Raj A, et al. Recruitment, promotion, and retention of women in academic medicine: how institutions are addressing gender disparities. Womens Health Issues 2017;27(3):374–81.
8. Kaplan SE, Raj A, Carr PL, et al. Race/ethnicity and success in academic medicine: findings from a longitudinal multi-institutional study. Acad Med 2018; 93(4):616.
9. ACGME. Specialty-specific References for DIOs: Program Director Qualifications [Internet]. Chicago (IL): Accreditation Council for Graduate Medical Education; 2019 July [updated 2019 Jul; cited 2020 Jul 12]. Available at: https://www.acgme.org/Portals/0/PDFs/Specialty-specific%20Requirement%20Topics/DIO-PD_Qualifications.pdf.
10. Al Achkar M, Hanauer M, Morrison EH, et al. Changing trends in residents-as-teachers across graduate medical education. Adv Med Educ Pract 2017;8:299.
11. Weinstein DF. Feedback in clinical education: untying the Gordian knot. Acad Med 2015;90(5):559–61.
12. Sullivan PB, Buckle A, Nicky G, et al. Peer observation of teaching as a faculty development tool. BMC Med Educ 2012;12(1):1–6.
13. Taylor DC, Hamdy H. Adult learning theories: Implications for learning and teaching in medical education: AMEE Guide No. 83. Med Teach 2013;35(11): e1561–72.
14. Sullivan GM. A toolkit for medical education scholarship. Journal of graduate medical education 2018;10(1):1.
15. Molloy E, Bearman M. Embracing the tension between vulnerability and credibility:'intellectual candour'in health professions education. Med Educ 2019;53(1): 32–41.

16. Grant J. Principles of curriculum design. Understanding medical education: evidence, theory and practice 2a. Malden: Wiley Blackwell; 2014. p. 31–46.

17. Barrows HS, Tamblyn RM. Problem-based learning: an approach to medical education, vol. 1. New York: Springer Publishing Company; 1980.

18. Koh GCH. Revisiting the 'Essentials of problem-based learning'. Med Education 2016;50(6):596–9.

19. Parmelee DX, Hudes P. Team-based learning: a relevant strategy in health professionals' education. Med Teach 2012;34(5):411–3.

20. McGaghie WC, Issenberg SB, Cohen MER, et al. Does simulation-based medical education with deliberate practice yield better results than traditional clinical education? A meta-analytic comparative review of the evidence. Acad Med 2011; 86(6):706.

21. Schuller MC, DaRosa DA, Crandall ML. Using just-in-time teaching and peer instruction in a residency program's core curriculum: enhancing satisfaction, engagement, and retention. Acad Med 2015;90(3):384–91.

22. Hew KF, Lo CK. Flipped classroom improves student learning in health professions education: a meta-analysis. BMC Med Educ 2018;18(1):38.

23. Gordon RJ. Launching your career in medical education [Internet]. Waltham (MA): Massachusetts Medical Society; 2017 Mar 16 [cited 2020 Jul 12]. Available from: https://resident360.nejm.org/expert-consult/launching-your-career-in-medical-education-3.

24. Pettit RK, McCoy L, Kinney M, et al. Student perceptions of gamified audience response system interactions in large group lectures and via lecture capture technology. BMC Med Educ 2015;15(1):92.

25. Wong G, Greenhalgh T, Pawson R. Internet-based medical education: a realist review of what works, for whom and in what circumstances. BMC Med Educ 2010;10(1):1–10.

26. Sharma N, Doherty I, Dong C. Adaptive learning in medical education: the final piece of technology enhanced learning? Ulster Med J 2017;86(3):198.

27. Guze PA. Using technology to meet the challenges of medical education. Trans Am Clin Climatol Assoc 2015;126:260.

28. Lockyer J, Carraccio C, Chan M-K, et al. Core principles of assessment in competency-based medical education. Med Teach 2017;39(6):609–16.

29. Swing SR, Cowley DS, Bentman A. Assessing resident performance on the psychiatry milestones. Acad Psychiatry 2014;38(3):294–302.

30. Boyce P, Spratt C, Davies M, et al. Using entrustable professional activities to guide curriculum development in psychiatry training. BMC Med Educ 2011; 11(1):96.

31. Steinert Y. The "problem" learner: whose problem is it? AMEE Guide No. 76. Med Teach 2013;35(4):e1035–45.

32. Coyle D. The culture code: the secrets of highly successful groups. New York: Bantam; 2018.

33. Adamson R, Goodman RB, Kritek P, et al. Training the teachers. The clinician-educator track of the university of Washington pulmonary and critical care medicine fellowship program. Ann Am Thorac Soc 2015;12(4):480–5.

34. Ahn J, Martin SK, Farnan JM, et al. The graduate medical education scholars track: developing residents as clinician–educators during clinical training via a longitudinal, multimodal, and multidisciplinary track. Acad Med 2018;93(2): 214–9.

35. Borges NJ, Navarro AM, Grover A, et al. How, when, and why do physicians choose careers in academic medicine? A literature review. Acad Med 2010; 85(4):680–6.
36. Colleges AoAM. Faculty roster. Washington, DC: U.S. Medical School Faculty; 2015.
37. U.S. Census Bureau QuickFacts: United States [Internet]. Census Bureau Quick-Facts. [cited 2020 Jul 12]. Available at: https://www.census.gov/quickfacts/fact/table/US/PST045219.
38. Sánchez NF, Rankin S, Callahan E, et al. LGBT trainee and health professional perspectives on academic careers—facilitators and challenges. LGBT health 2015;2(4):346–56.
39. Sheikh MH, Chaudhary AMD, Khan AS, et al. Influences for gender disparity in academic psychiatry in the United States. Cureus 2018;10(4):e2514.
40. Pololi LH, Krupat E, Civian JT, et al. Why are a quarter of faculty considering leaving academic medicine? A study of their perceptions of institutional culture and intentions to leave at 26 representative US medical schools. Acad Med 2012; 87(7):859–69.
41. Chaudhary AMD, Naveed S, Siddiqi J, et al. US psychiatry faculty: academic rank, gender and racial profile. Acad Psychiatry 2020;44(3):260–6.
42. Nelson A. Unequal treatment: confronting racial and ethnic disparities in health care. J Natl Med Assoc 2002;94(8):666.

Neuroscience Education
Making It Relevant to Psychiatric Training

Check for
updates

Joseph J. Cooper, MD[a],*, Ashley E. Walker, MD[b]

KEYWORDS

- Neuroscience • Education • Psychiatry • Neuropsychiatry

KEY POINTS

- Neuroscience perspectives integrate alongside other traditional psychiatric perspectives.
- Neuroscience education is most effective when it is case-based, clinically relevant, interactive, informed by adult learning theory, and fun!
- Neuroscience education must be individualized to the needs of the learner(s).
- Lessons from neuropsychiatry can help us to better understand our patients' brain function at the bedside.
- Integrating neuroscience perspectives means integrating the pathophysiology of our diseases, and thus is essential for the field of psychiatry to take its proper place in modern medicine.

INTRODUCTION

Modern medicine is grounded in the scientific application of evidence-based treatments that target the pathophysiology of disease. Yet, in psychiatry we have struggled to move past a dualistic separation of mind from brain, and to embrace our identity as a clinical neuroscience discipline.[1] As a product of this implicit dualism, our educational systems have treated neuroscience as, at most, a topic among many others given an hourly didactic slot for an academic quarter or so. To truly join our colleagues in modern medicine, we must integrate a neuroscience perspective into all aspects of psychiatric education and practice.

However, barriers to the integration of neuroscience perspectives remain (**Table 1**). Much of clinical psychiatry today involves making evidence-based decisions based on clinical symptom checklists, all of which can be done without bringing attention to the underlying pathophysiology. In other medical fields, this type of practice is theoretically possible (eg, the prescription of antiarrhythmic agents for a particular cardiac syndrome without being able to consider the electrical circuitry of the heart), but would

[a] Department of Psychiatry, University of Illinois at Chicago, Chicago, IL, USA; [b] Department of Psychiatry, University of Oklahoma School of Community Medicine, 4502 East 41st Street, Tulsa, OK 74135, USA
* Corresponding author. 912 South Wood Street (MC 913), Chicago, IL 60612.
E-mail address: cooperj@uic.edu

Psychiatr Clin N Am 44 (2021) 295–307
https://doi.org/10.1016/j.psc.2020.12.008
0193-953X/21/© 2020 Elsevier Inc. All rights reserved.

psych.theclinics.com

Table 1
Challenges to making neuroscience relevant in undergraduate, graduate, and continuing medical education

General Challenges to Integrating Neuroscience into Psychiatric Education		
Unsure where to start or what to cover		
Lack of interested, qualified, and effective teachers		
Lack of integration into clinical settings		
Lack of time		
Undergraduate Medical Education Specific	**Graduate Medical Education Specific**	**Continuing Medical Education Specific**
Implicit dualism – students see psychiatry services often physically separated from other medical services	Perceived lack of resident interest	Older psychiatric workforce
	Engaging diverse stakeholders (researchers, clinical educators)	Rapid growth of psychiatric neuroscience content in the last quarter century
Historic stereotypes of psychoanalytic settings	Limited time for outside reading	Lifetime certificates issued by the American Board of Psychiatry and Neurology until 1994
Not seeing psychiatry as a scientific discipline or "real" medicine	Lack of assessment tools	Brain is perceived as an "unknow-able" black box (remnants of dualism)

be considered a strange and unscientific approach to practice. A patient-centered discussion of pathophysiology is typical in modern medicine, and can help patient comfort and buy-in to the treatment plan. Many calls for the neuroscience revolution in clinical psychiatry[1–3] have been followed up by a variety of practical recommendations for how this can be done.[4–7] It begins with our educational systems.

Although the term "psychiatric neuroscience" often invokes thoughts of cutting-edge research and the development of futuristic diagnostic procedures, there is much about our patients' brain function that is readily knowable today. Better yet, this information is already available in every psychiatric patient encounter. However, a psychiatric physical examination is often omitted or incomplete,[8–17] and cognitive examination, when done, rarely extends beyond a standardized screening tool such as the Mini Mental State Examination[18] or the Montreal Cognitive Assessment,[19] and thus fails to fully inform the clinician about the function of behaviorally relevant cortical and subcortical networks.[20] Challenges to the integration of neuroscience[7,21,22] are discussed in this article and summarized in **Table 1**.

UNDERGRADUATE MEDICAL EDUCATION CHALLENGES

Undergraduate medical education is an opportunity to frame expectations about the integration of neuroscience and clinical psychiatry. The historic lack of this integration likely contributes to psychiatry's difficulty in attracting undergraduate neuroscience majors into the field.[23] One major influence on how medical students understand the larger world of medicine is the United States Medical Licensing Exam. Unfortunately, the United States Medical Licensing Exam still reinforces a dualistic perspective: in their examination's content outline[24] there are separate sections for "Behavioral Health," which includes most major categories of psychiatric disorders, and "Nervous System & Special Senses," which includes many disorders that typically involve psychiatric evaluation and management, including delirium, fibromyalgia, primary insomnia, tic disorders, neuroleptic malignant syndrome, and neurodegenerative disorders. This selective parsing of only some neuropsychiatric disorders into nervous system diseases leaves our students at best confused, and at worst, with the impression that other psychiatric disorders do not have a brain-based etiology.

The Association of Directors of Medical Student Education in Psychiatry has developed Learning Goals and Milestones for all undergraduate medical student education in psychiatry.[25] These goals consist of six categories of learning goals, divided into preclinical and clinical education, with a total of 70 individual items for students to master. Overall, there is very little mention of neurobiology or pathophysiology. The prefix "neuro" appears only once in the 70 items: "Describe the neurobiological basis of the substance use disorders, and indicate both intoxication and withdrawal syndromes." The other item mentioning pathophysiology states: "Describe the psychobiological-behavioral models for the major psychiatric disorders." It is not clear whether the differential wording is intentional, but it may leave learners with the impression that neurobiology has minimal relevance to major psychiatric disorders.

Additionally, other Association of Directors of Medical Student Education in Psychiatry items imply a dualistic perspective of mind/body separation including: "apply knowledge of the expected changes across the lifespan in the care of patients with psychiatric disorders and medical conditions" and "prioritize a differential diagnosis by applying knowledge of psychopathology and medical illnesses." This phrasing implies that psychiatric disorders and psychopathology are not medical conditions or illnesses, and could be easily remedied by adding the word "other" before the word medical, to indicate that "psychiatric disorders" are 1 subtype of "medical conditions." This approach was taken with the *Diagnostic and Statistical Manual of Mental Disorders*, 5th edition,[26] whereby psychiatric disorders were recognized as being possibly caused by "another medical condition," implying that the idiopathic psychiatric disorder is also a medical condition. With regard to neuropsychiatric evaluation, there is no specific mention of psychiatric physical examination skills in the Association of Directors of Medical Student Education in Psychiatry Learning Goals and Milestones. Finally, although we applaud the specific mention of cognitive testing in the item, "demonstrate ability to perform a cognitive screening," the focus is on using a screening tool, rather than the use of cognitive testing to localize functioning versus dysfunctioning neural systems.

GRADUATE MEDICAL EDUCATION CHALLENGES

Psychiatric residency programs have not sufficiently integrated neuroscience perspectives into training, a point agreed upon by residents and fellows,[27] chief residents,[28] program directors,[21] department chairs,[29] and practicing psychiatrists.[29] It was not until the official release of The Psychiatry Milestones Project[30] in 2015 that the word "neuroscience" appeared anywhere in the training expectations for psychiatry. A second edition of Psychiatry Milestones was published in March 2020,[31] and is due to take effect July 1, 2021. This second edition sets a much higher bar for the integration of neuroscience into clinical care. As an example, whereas the first edition held at level 4 (the expected level for a graduating psychiatry resident) that a resident "explains neurobiological hypotheses and genetic risks of common psychiatric disorders to patients," now it is expected that a resident "correlates neurobiological processes into case formulation and treatment planning." As a field, we are ready to move away from calling all of neuroscience "hypotheses" and toward a practice wherein we can honestly interact with that which is known about the neurobiology of psychiatric disorders, while acknowledging the areas that remain to be understood.

CONTINUING MEDICAL EDUCATION CHALLENGES

To make neuroscience education relevant to psychiatric training, it has to first be relevant to the trainers. One of the central barriers in highlighting the salience of neuroscience education for trainees is the dearth of faculty who feel comfortable teaching it. Most psychiatrists are over the age of 55[32] and graduated residency by the early 1990s. At that time, the neuroscience revolution was celebrating the mapping of the sequence of the gene for Huntington's disease. The rapid expansion of neuroscience discoveries in the last 25 years is compounded by the tradition of the American Board of Psychiatry and Neurology to issue lifetime certificates until 1994.[33] Psychiatrists certified before then have no American Board of Psychiatry and Neurology requirements to learn additional information, ever. Absent this external motivation, it remains incumbent upon practitioners to find their own internal motivation to keep pace with the exponential growth in neuroscience discoveries that are redefining how we think about the brain, mental illness, and treatment.

SOLUTIONS

Organized efforts to advance neuroscience education include published single-institution curricula,[34–40] reviews of previously published curricula,[41] and textbooks, some of which have taken a more accessible[42] and others a more comprehensive approach.[43] Here, we review and highlight 3 major efforts to bring neuroscience perspectives to education and practice, the National Neuroscience Curriculum Initiative (NNCI), neuroscience-based nomenclature (NbN), and lessons from neuropsychiatry.

The National Neuroscience Curriculum Initiative

The NNCI arose in 2013 through collaboration with the American Association of Directors of Psychiatric Residency Training and has been supported by the National Institute for Mental Health, American Association of Directors of Psychiatric Residency Training, the Society of Biological Psychiatry, and the American College of Neuropsychopharmacology.[7] The NNCI is an open-access educational initiative and e-learning repository for peer-reviewed resources for teaching psychiatric neuroscience whose learning objectives include that: "(1) Participants will appreciate the importance of neuroscience to the future of psychiatry and to the way we will approach patient care; (2) Participants will demonstrate an understanding of core concepts in neuroscience, including how complex interactions between environmental stressors and disruptions in neural circuitry may contribute to different psychiatric disorders; and (3) Participants will be able to serve as ambassadors of neuroscience who can thoughtfully communicate findings from the field to professional and lay audiences."[7]

The NNCI has hosted the American Association of Directors of Psychiatric Residency Training premeeting 7 times from 2014 to 2020, with 160 to 240 attendees each year, and more than 90% of participants have indicated that they were likely or very likely to implement at least one of the demonstrated approaches.[7] In addition to presenting at sponsoring organizations' annual meetings, the NNCI has given educational presentations at the annual meetings of the Academy for Consultation-Liaison Psychiatry, the American Academy of Child and Adolescent Psychiatry, the American Psychiatric Association, the Association for Academic Psychiatry, and the Association of American Medical Colleges, and presented grand rounds at universities across the United States, and internationally in Canada, Brazil, the UK (in collaboration with the Royal College of Psychiatry), the Netherlands, Mozambique, and South Africa. The NNCI's reach into graduate medical education has been extensive: more than 200 US psychiatry residency and fellowship training programs have reported integration of NNCI materials into their educational programs.[7] The NNCI has made an international impact as well: between March 2015 and June 2019, the website (www.nncionline.org) hosted 48,640 unique users from 161 countries with 500,953 page views.[7]

It is imperative that psychiatric trainees develop attitudes and practices that embrace the necessity for life-long learning, in general and especially as it relates to neuroscience, as this field continues to rapidly grow and transform.[44] The philosophic approach of the NNCI has been informed by adult learning theory to keep the information approachable, accessible, and fun for learners, with the hope that this engagement will excite trainees to want to learn more.[7]

To reinforce the importance of neuroscience to patient care, the NNCI's "Neuroscience Lab" sessions revolve around clinical cases or real-life scenarios while capitalizing on multimodal sensory learning. These sessions include a variety of interactive approaches, such as drawing, play dough construction, collage making, and playing games.[7] Both online and classroom-based Neuroscience Lab modules are available to fit the needs of either programs or individuals. For example, exercises such as Truth or Dare: Chronic Pain[45] include friendly competition as a motivator for learning, whereas in the Find It, Draw It, Know It sessions,[46] learners may follow along with a video to practice drawing neural pathways on their own as often as they need.

Similarly, other NNCI content seeks to engage the learner where they are, literally and figuratively. Recognizing that much of education actually occurs outside the classroom, the NNCI developed session frameworks specifically intended to be used in clinical settings. By bridging the gap between the classroom and the clinic, Clinical Neuroscience Conversations bring an understanding of neuroscience to the day-to-day practice of psychiatry.[47] In these sessions, participants review and discuss a typical clinical case (such as borderline personality disorder[48] or functional neurologic symptom disorder[49]) with their team, then watch a brief video explaining a salient neuroscience concept that alters or enhances the way they would typically formulate the case. They then discuss the new information and apply it to the original case to enrich the formulation or treatment plan. Using a similar format, a subset of these modules—Talking Pathways to Patients—have participants role-play an explanation of the neurobiology to a patient.[7,50,51] Participants are thus able to not only see the clinical relevance of the neurobiology, but also gain practice using it to enhance patient care. By providing the case, video, and discussion questions for these modules, these materials address numerous potential barriers to neuroscience integration (as in **Table 1**), such as lack of curricular time, lack of qualified teachers, and lack of reading time, and directly engage both learners and faculty.

Given that a lack of qualified faculty is the largest perceived barrier to increasing training in neuroscience and neuropsychiatry,[21] even with ready-made sessions and full facilitator's guides, many faculty may feel inadequate when it comes to teaching neuroscience. A busy clinical faculty member who was not themselves exposed to quality neuroscience education during training may not appreciate the relevance of neuroscience to current care. Yet it is critical to engage these faculty, because they are the ones who have to educate and influence psychiatric trainees.

The barriers to engaging clinician educators and getting them up to speed with neuroscience are the same as those encountered with trainees. Faculty time is precious, and activities aimed at their own education need to be made as clinically relevant and time efficient as possible, while still using principles of adult learning. Nearly all of the NNCI's content can be easily adapted for faculty education: Clinical Neuroscience Conversations and Talking Pathways to Patients sessions can be viewed and reviewed individually. So too can the Neuroscience in the Media, Progressive Case Conference, Integrative Case Conference, and Translational Neuroscience classroom sessions be used as self-study materials through application of the facilitator's guides.

Additionally, the NNCI's "What to Say When Patients Ask" modules in particular were designed to deliver high-yield content to faculty in a manner that emphasizes the clinical relevance of the neuroscience material.[52] These sessions start by reviewing a brief clinical scenario and practicing role playing answering a patient's questions about their illness, symptoms, or treatment. Participants then read or watch a brief Clinical Commentary article or video and discuss its key take home points. They then practice role playing a second time, incorporating their newfound neuroscience perspective to enhance their answers to the patient.[7] Although still applicable to resident psychiatrists, the What to Say When Patients Ask is a format that can also be used in a faculty development setting to engage multiple faculty simultaneously. More than 45 such Clinical Commentaries have been published by the NNCI in the journal *Biological Psychiatry* and these commentaries were 3 of the top 30 most downloaded articles of the journal in both 2017 and 2018.[7]

For particularly reluctant faculty, incentives from both "above" and "below" may help them to appreciate the relevance of neuroscience to current practice. From above, the American Board of Psychiatry and Neurology's recently developed Maintenance of Certification Pilot Program includes several articles with clear neuroscience themes.[53–57] This indicates that regulatory bodies are already emphasizing the relevance of neuroscience to ongoing psychiatric education and current clinical practice. Additionally, energy from below, in the form of trainees eager to learn and incorporate new neuroscience knowledge, may motivate psychiatric educators to incorporate more neuroscience concepts into both didactic materials and clinical practice.[27,28]

To maintain the most relevance, educational materials must fit or be adapted to changing needs and trends. The coronavirus disease-2019 pandemic precipitated a rapid educational shift into online or other virtual learning formats, for both self-study and group and classroom activities. Educators at all levels were tasked with creating or reformatting their curriculum to work around the time and physical constraints of learners who could no longer attend regular classroom activities as well as lecturers who similarly could no longer present materials in a traditional format.[58] Although online learning is not a new concept,[59] its incorporation into medical education has been slow; the pandemic served as a catalyst for more people to use, develop, and disseminate additional innovative teaching materials. In response to these learner needs, the NNCI developed and disseminated a 14-day "Quarantine Curriculum" that incorporates both self-study activities as well as interactive, real-time learning experiences.[58,60] Although it was designed with the needs of psychiatry residents and fellows in mind, the curriculum captured an even broader audience, ranging from medical students to researchers, suggesting that it is difficult to determine a priori who will find a given educational tool most relevant.

One challenging area that remains, which is a key issue for residency training programs, is the development of comprehensive neuroscience curriculum. In other, more established areas of psychiatry, it may be easier for individual programs to develop educational materials with minimal direction. For example, regarding psychotherapy training, the ACGME Program Requirements for psychiatry provide only 2 instructions: that residents must demonstrate competence in managing patients with "concurrent use of medications and psychotherapy," and have experience in the "initial evaluation and treatment of ongoing individual psychotherapy patients, some of whom should be seen weekly."[61] Despite this lack of explicit direction, program directors and psychotherapy educators may still feel comfortable with and capable of providing comprehensive psychotherapy training. Presumably this is because they received training in psychotherapy themselves, there are readily available, authoritative textbooks in this area, and the material itself is established and relatively unchanged since they trained. However, for neuroscience training, these benefits often do not apply.

Just as it would be impossible to create a single psychotherapy curriculum that suits the needs of every program and individual learner, so too is it impossible to create a one-size-fits-all neuroscience curriculum. Instead, the NNCI has worked to create a myriad of resources that can be adapted to individuals' needs and provided samples of various ways in which their materials might be used.[22] The NNCI also offers individual programs the opportunity for a consultation to build or enhance their own neuroscience curricula, by performing a Strengths, Weaknesses, Opportunities, and Threats (SWOT) analysis and customizing a set of curricular options to suit the program's unique needs and resources.[7] The ability to personalize curricular content helps to maximize the relevance of neuroscience at the level of the program.

Neuroscience-Based Nomenclature

Our current method of classifying psychotropic medications—for example, antidepressants, antipsychotics, mood stabilizers, and so on—fails to account for differences in mechanism of action, or even the usage of the medication (eg, the use of "antipsychotics" for treating psychosis, mood disorders, agitation in delirium, and other conditions). This process can be confusing for trainees as well as patients, potentially stigmatizing, and unhelpful for a clinician trying to make an informed choice regarding the next pharmacologic trial.[62–64]

In 2008, 5 international scientific organizations—the European College of Neuropsychopharmacology, the American College of Neuropsychopharmacology, the International College of Neuropsychopharmacology, the Asian College of Neuropsychopharmacology, and the International Union of Basic and Clinical Pharmacology—established a task force to develop a new, pharmacologically driven system for naming psychotropic medications.[63] What they came up with was the NbN (nbn2r.com), the second edition of which now includes 130 medications.[65] The NbN represents a rational nomenclature that is based on contemporary knowledge, helpful in making clinical decisions, not in conflict with the use of medications, and capable of accommodating new compounds.[63,65] The NbN also includes information on approved indications, efficacy and side effects, practical clinical knowledge, and neurobiology.[62,63] For example, instead of just referring to the "antipsychotic" risperidone, NbN denotes this medication as a dopamine, serotonin, and norepinephrine antagonist and describes its usefulness in schizophrenia, bipolar disorder, and other conditions. NbN also helps highlight for learners that some of our commonly used medication categories already have logical names, based on mechanism of action (eg, selective serotonin reuptake inhibitors), whereas others have names based on their molecular structure and/or one of their many clinical indications (eg, tricyclic antidepressants). By the end of 2016, several leading neuroscience journals agreed to use the NbN when referring to medications in their publications.[63,64,66–68]

By providing clinically useful information in an easily accessible format (online or mobile application), NbN makes psychopharmacological neuroscience relevant to health care professionals at all levels—undergraduate, graduate, and continuing medical education.[65] To maintain relevance and accuracy, the NbN taskforce plans to update the NbN twice per year. The app also includes a feature by which to provide feedback and suggestions, in this way engaging the end user as a key stakeholder in integrating neuroscience into clinical or training settings.

Lessons from Neuropsychiatry

If we are to integrate neuroscience perspectives into psychiatric education, we must start with the neuroscience information obtainable at the bedside and in the clinic: the physical neurologic examination, including testing cognitive function. This allows us to develop behaviorally relevant differential diagnoses which consider idiopathic psychiatric categories, such as bipolar mania, along with other neurologic or systemic medical conditions, such as seizure disorder, frontotemporal dementia, or autoimmune encephalitis. Beyond the freely available bedside tools, basic neurodiagnostic tests including electroencephalography,[69–72] brain imaging,[73–76] and lumbar puncture[77,78] have a range of behavioral indications yet are widely underemphasized in psychiatric education and underused in clinical psychiatric settings. The American Neuropsychiatric Association issued guidelines on Neuropsychiatry Training Objectives for General Psychiatry Residents in 2001.[79] And although nearly 20 years old, they continue to set a high bar for the incorporation of neurologic examination, neurodiagnostic interpretation, and neuroanatomic localization skills in addition to knowledge of diagnosis and treatment of a wide range of neuropsychiatric disorders. These guidelines serve as a reminder that, even if neuroscience is more relevant to psychiatric education in 2020, it has always been relevant, as our diseases are diseases of the brain.

SUMMARY

Psychiatry is neuroscience. From the doctor–patient relationship to psychotherapy to housing initiatives to psychopharmacology to deep brain stimulation, all psychiatric interventions are neuroscience-based interventions. The complexity of the brain is one of many factors that have impeded our field's acknowledgment and embracement of our target organ. The practice of modern psychiatry requires the inclusion of neuroscience perspectives in every facet of our work. But rather than a daunting task, embracing the brain, acquiring neuroscience knowledge, and incorporating it into our practices can be engaging, exciting, and fun.

CLINICS CARE POINTS

- Neuroscience perspectives integrate alongside other traditional psychiatric perspectives.
- Neuroscience education is most effective when it is case-based, clinically relevant, interactive, informed by adult learning theory, and fun!
- Neuroscience education must be individualized to the needs of the learner(s).
- Lessons from neuropsychiatry can help us to better understand our patients' brain function at the bedside.
- Integrating neuroscience perspectives means integrating the pathophysiology of our diseases, and thus is essential for the field of psychiatry to take its proper place in modern medicine.

DISCLOSURE

The authors have nothing to disclose.

REFERENCES

1. Insel TR, Quirion R. Psychiatry as a clinical neuroscience discipline. JAMA 2005; 294(17):2221–4.

2. Akil M, Etkin A. Transforming neuroscience education in psychiatry. Acad Psychiatry 2014;38(2):116–20.
3. Arbuckle MR, Travis MJ, Ross DA. Integrating a neuroscience perspective into clinical psychiatry today. JAMA Psychiatry 2017;74(4):313–4.
4. Torous J, Stern AP, Padmanabhan JL, et al. A proposed solution to integrating cognitive-affective neuroscience and neuropsychiatry in psychiatry residency training: the time is now. Asian J Psychiatr 2015;17:116–21.
5. Schildkrout B, Benjamin S, Lauterbach MD. Integrating neuroscience knowledge and neuropsychiatric skills into psychiatry: the way forward. Acad Med 2016; 91(5):650–6.
6. Cooper JJ, Korb AS, Akil M. Bringing neuroscience to the bedside. Focus 2019; 17(1):2–7.
7. Arbuckle MR, Travis MJ, Eisen J, et al. Transforming psychiatry from the classroom to the clinic: lessons from the National Neuroscience Curriculum Initiative. Acad Psychiatry 2020;44(1):29–36.
8. Menninger KA. A manual for psychiatric case study. 2nd edition. New York: Grune & Stratton; 1962. p. 48–9.
9. McIntyre JS, Romano J. Is there a stethoscope in the house (and is it used)? Arch Gen Psychiatry 1977;34(10):1147–51.
10. Krummel S, Kathol RG. What you should know about physical evaluations in psychiatric patients: results of a survey. Gen Hosp Psychiatry 1987;9(4):275–9.
11. Rigby JC, Oswald AG. An evaluation of the performing and recording of physical examinations by psychiatric trainees. Br J Psychiatry 1987;150(04):533–5.
12. Hodgson R, Adeyemo O. Physical examination performed by psychiatrists. Int J Psychiatry Clin Pract 2004;8(1):57–60.
13. Vanezis AP, Manns D. Physical examinations of mental health service users. Prog Neurol Psychiatry 2010;14(4):19–23.
14. Murray J, Baillon S. Case series of physical examinations on psychiatric inpatients: influence of a structured form on the quality of documentation. J Ment Health 2013;22(5):428–38.
15. Murray J, Baillon S, Bruce J, et al. A survey of psychiatrists' attitudes towards the physical examination. J Ment Health 2015;24(4):249–54.
16. Azzam PN, Gopalan P, Brown JR, et al. Physical examination for the academic psychiatrist: primer and common clinical scenarios. Acad Psychiatry 2016; 40(2):321–7.
17. Medina M, Garza DM, Cooper JJ. Physical examination skills among chief residents in psychiatry: practices, attitudes, and self-perceived knowledge. Acad Psychiatry 2020;44(1):68–72.
18. Folstein MF, Folstein SE, McHugh PR. Mini-Mental State: a practical method for grading the cognitive state of patients for the clinician. J Psychiatr Res 1975; 12:189–98.
19. Nasreddine ZS, Phillips NA, Bédirian V, et al. The Montreal Cognitive Assessment, MoCA: a brief screening tool for mild cognitive impairment. J Am Geriatr Soc 2005;53(4):695–9.
20. Benjamin S, Lauterbach MD. The neurological examination adapted for neuropsychiatry. CNS Spectr 2018;23(3):219–27.
21. Benjamin S, Travis MJ, Cooper JJ, et al. Neuropsychiatry and neuroscience education of psychiatry trainees: attitudes and barriers. Acad Psychiatry 2014; 38(2):135–40.

22. Walker A, Kotara S, Pershern L, et al. Incorporating NNCI resources into a curriculum. 2019. Available at: https://www.nncionline.org/course/incorporating-nnci-resources-into-a-curriculum/. Accessed April 10, 2020.

23. Goldenberg MN, Krystal JH. Undergraduate neuroscience majors: a missed opportunity for psychiatry workforce development. Acad Psychiatry 2017;41(2): 239–42.

24. The Federation of State Medical Boards of the United States, Inc., and the National Board of Medical Examiners. USMLE Content Outline. 2020. Available at: https://www.usmle.org/pdfs/usmlecontentoutline.pdf. Accessed April 24, 2020.

25. The Association of Directors of Medical Student Education in Psychiatry. Learning goals and milestones. 2020. Available at: https://www.admsep.org/milestones.php?c=learning-goals. Accessed April 28, 2020.

26. American Psychiatric Association. Diagnostic and statistical manual of mental disorders: diagnostic and statistical manual of mental disorders. 5th edition. Arlington (VA): American Psychiatric Association; 2013.

27. Fung LK, Akil M, Widge A, et al. Attitudes toward neuroscience education among psychiatry residents and fellows. Acad Psychiatry 2014;38(2):127–34.

28. Bennett JI, Handa K, Mahajan A, et al. Psychiatry chief resident opinions toward basic and clinical neuroscience training and practice. Acad Psychiatry 2014; 38(2):141–4.

29. Fung LK, Akil M, Widge A, et al. Attitudes toward neuroscience education in psychiatry: a national multi-stakeholder survey. Acad Psychiatry 2015;39(2):139–46.

30. The Accreditation Council for Graduate Medical Education and The American Board of Psychiatry and Neurology. The Psychiatry Milestone Project. 2015. Available at: https://www.acgme.org/Portals/0/PDFs/Milestones/PsychiatryMilestones.pdf. Accessed April 27, 2020.

31. The Accreditation Council for Graduate Medical Education. Psychiatry Milestones. 2020. Available at: https://www.acgme.org/Portals/0/PDFs/Milestones/PsychiatryMilestones2.0.pdf. Accessed April 27, 2020.

32. Association of American Medical Colleges. Active physicians by age and specialty. 2015. Available at: https://www.aamc.org/data-reports/workforce/interactive-data/active-physicians-age-and-specialty-2015. Accessed April 25, 2020.

33. The American Board of Psychiatry and Neurology, Inc. Lifetime certificate holders. Available at: https://www.abpn.com/maintain-certification/maintenance-of-certification-program/lifetime-certificate-holders/. Accessed April 28, 2020.

34. Lacy T, Hughes JD. A neural systems-based neurobiology and neuropsychiatry course: integrating biology, psychodynamics, and psychology in the psychiatric curriculum. Acad Psychiatry 2006;30:410–5.

35. Dunstone DC. Neurosciences-in-psychiatry curriculum project for residents in psychiatry. Acad Psychiatry 2010;34:31–8.

36. Etkin A, Cuthbert B. Beyond the DSM: development of a transdiagnostic psychiatric neuroscience course. Acad Psychiatry 2014;38(2):145–50.

37. Griffith JL. Neuroscience and humanistic psychiatry: a residency curriculum. Acad Psychiatry 2014;38(2):177–84.

38. Gopalan P, Azzam PN, Travis MJ, et al. Longitudinal interdisciplinary neuroscience curriculum. Acad Psychiatry 2014;38(2):163–7.

39. Ross DA, Rohrbaugh R. Integrating neuroscience in the training of psychiatrists: a patient-centered didactic curriculum based on adult learning principles. Acad Psychiatry 2014;38(2):154–62.

40. Cookey J, Butterfield M, Robichaud C, et al. Integrating clinical neurosciences in a psychiatry residency training program: a brief report with pilot data. Acad Psychiatry 2018;42(2):217–21.
41. Coverdale J, Balon R, Beresin EV, et al. Teaching clinical neuroscience to psychiatry residents: model curricula. Acad Psychiatry 2014;38(2):111–5.
42. Higgins ES, George MS. The neuroscience of clinical psychiatry: the pathophysiology of behavior and mental illness. 3rd edition. Philadelphia: Lippincott Williams & Wilkins; 2018.
43. Charney DS, Buxbaum JD, Sklar P, et al. Neurobiology of mental illness. 5th edition. New York: Oxford University Press; 2018.
44. Yeung AWK, Goto TK, Leung WK. The changing landscape of neuroscience research, 2006-2015: a bibliometric study. Front Neurosci 2017;11:120.
45. Baller E. Truth or dare: chronic pain. 2020. National Neuroscience Curriculum Initiative. Available at: https://www.nncionline.org/course/truth-or-dare-chronic-pain/. Accessed April 29, 2020.
46. White R. Find it, draw it, know it: fear circuitry. National Neuroscience Curriculum Initiative. 2016. Available at: https://www.nncionline.org/course/find-it-draw-it-know-it/. Accessed April 29, 2020.
47. Ross D, Arbuckle M, Wang A, et al. Facilitator's guide: clinical neuroscience conversations. National Neuroscience Curriculum Initiative. 2016. Available at: https://www.nncionline.org/wp-content/uploads/2016/03/CNC_FacilitatorsGuide_p6.pdf. Accessed April 29, 2020.
48. Epigenetics and trauma. National Neuroscience Curriculum Initiative. Available at: https://www.nncionline.org/course/epigenetics/. Accessed May 1, 2020.
49. Madva E, Cooper JJ. Functional neurological disorder. National Neuroscience Curriculum Initiative. 2018. Available at: https://www.nncionline.org/course/functional-neurological-disorder/. Accessed April 29, 2020.
50. Karampahtsis C, Travis M, Arbuckle M. Talking pathways to patients: addiction. National Neuroscience Curriculum Initiative. Available at: https://www.nncionline.org/course/talking-pathways-to-patients-addiction/. Accessed April 29, 2020.
51. Jibson M. Talking pathways to patients: borderline personality disorder. National Neuroscience Curriculum Initiative. 2017. Available at: https://www.nncionline.org/course/talking-pathways-to-patients-borderline-personality-disorder/. Accessed April 29, 2020.
52. What to Say When Patients Ask. National Neuroscience Curriculum Initiative. Available at: https://www.nncionline.org/what-to-say-when-patients-ask/. Accessed April 29, 2020.
53. Volkow ND, Boyle M. Neuroscience of addiction: relevance to prevention and treatment. Am J Psychiatry 2018;175(8):729–40.
54. Sanacora G, Frye MA, McDonald W, et al. A consensus statement on the use of ketamine in the treatment of mood disorders. JAMA Psychiatry 2017;74(4):399–405.
55. Brunet A, Saumier D, Liu A, et al. Reduction of PTSD symptoms with pre-reactivation propranolol therapy: a randomized controlled trial. Am J Psychiatry 2018;175(5):427–33.
56. Taber KH, Lindstrom CM, Hurley RA. Neural substrates of antisocial personality disorder: current state and future directions. J Neuropsychiatry Clin Neurosci 2016;28(4):256–61.
57. Ahmed RM, Paterson RW, Warren JD, et al. Biomarkers in dementia: clinical utility and new directions. J Neurol Neurosurg Psychiatry 2014;85(12):1426–34.

58. Ross DA. Creating a "Quarantine Curriculum" to enhance teaching and learning during the COVID-19 pandemic. Acad Med 2020. https://doi.org/10.1097/ACM.0000000000003424.

59. Ruiz JG, Mintzer MJ, Leipzig RM. The impact of e-learning in medical education. Acad Med 2006;81:207–12.

60. National Neuroscience Curriculum Initiative Quarantine Curriculum Committee. NNCI quarantine curriculum. 2020. Available at: https://www.nncionline.org/nnci-quarantine-curriculum/. Accessed April 19, 2020.

61. The Accreditation Council for Graduate Medical Education. ACGME program requirements for graduate medical education in psychiatry. 2019. Available at: https://www.acgme.org/Portals/0/PFAssets/ProgramRequirements/400_Psychiatry_2019.pdf. Accessed April 29, 2020.

62. Zohar J, Kasper S. Neuroscience-based nomenclature (NbN): a call for action. World J Biol Psychiatry 2016;17(5):318–20.

63. Möller HJ, Schmitt A, Falkai P. Neuroscience-based nomenclature (jNbN) to replace traditional terminology of psychotropic medications. Eur Arch Psychiatry Clin Neurosci 2016;266:385–6.

64. Krystal JH, Abi-Dargham A, Barch DM, et al. Biological psychiatry and biological psychiatry: cognitive neuroscience and neuroimaging adopt neuroscience-based nomenclature. Biol Psychiatry 2016;7(1):300–1.

65. NbN2r: neuroscience-based nomenclature, second edition-revised. 2017. Available at: http://nbn2r.com. Accessed April 27, 2020.

66. Frazer A, Blier P. A neuroscience-based nomenclature (NbN) for psychotropic agents. Int J Neuropsychopharmacol 2016;19(8):1–2.

67. Uchida H, Yamawaki S, Bahk WM, et al. Neuroscience-based nomenclature (NbN) for clinical psychopharmacology and neuroscience. Clin Psychopharmacol Neurosci 2016;14(2):115–6.

68. Nutt DJ, Blier P. Neuroscience-based nomenclature (NbN) for Journal of Psychopharmacology. J Psychopharmacol 2016;30(5):413–5.

69. Sand T, Bjørk MH, Vaaler AE. Is EEG a useful test in adult psychiatry? Tidsskr Nor Laegeforen 2013;133(11):1200–4.

70. Swatzyna RJ, Tarnow JD, Turner RP, et al. Integration of EEG into psychiatric practice: a step toward precision medicine for autism spectrum disorder. J Clin Neurophysiol 2017;34(3):230–5.

71. Hughes JR. A review of the usefulness of the standard EEG in psychiatry. Clin Electroencephalogr 1996;27(1):35–9.

72. Boutros NN. The forsaking of the clinical EEG by psychiatry: how justified? CNS Spectr 2018;23(3):196–204.

73. Medina M, Lee D, Garza DM, et al. Neuroimaging education in psychiatry residency training: needs assessment. Acad Psychiatry 2020;44(3):311–5.

74. Silbersweig DA, Rauch SL. Neuroimaging in psychiatry: a quarter century of progress. Harv Rev Psychiatry 2017;25(5):195.

75. Downar J, Krizova A, Ghaffar O, et al. Neuroimaging week: a novel, engaging, and effective curriculum for teaching neuroimaging to junior psychiatric residents. Acad Psychiatry 2010;34(2):119–24.

76. Barron DS. Magnetic resonance imaging for psychiatry. 2015. Available at: http://www.nncionline.org/course/magnetic-resonance-imaging-for-psychiatry/. Accessed April 25, 2020.

77. Pollak TA, Lennox BR. Time for a change of practice: the real-world value of testing for neuronal autoantibodies in acute first-episode psychosis. BJPsych Open 2018;4(4):262–4.

78. Shaw LM, Arias J, Blennow K, et al. Appropriate use criteria for lumbar puncture and cerebrospinal fluid testing in the diagnosis of Alzheimer's disease. Alzheimers Dement 2018;14(11):1505–21.

79. Benjamin S, Duffy J, Fogel B, et al. Neuropsychiatry training objectives for general psychiatry residents. American Neuropsychiatric Association; 2001. Available at: http://www.anpaonline.org/neuropsychiatry-training-objectives-for-general-psychiatryresidents. Accessed June 22, 2013.

Lifelong Learning in Psychiatry and the Role of Certification

Joan M. Anzia, MD[1]

KEYWORDS

• Lifelong learning • Board certification • Continuing education synopsis

KEY POINTS

• The key period of development of medical specialties occurred in the first half of the twentieth century, along with the development of certifying boards under the American Board of Medical Specialties (ABMS).

• The ABMS, in response to multiple stakeholders, rapid scientific and technological innovation, and other factors, began to mandate a continuing certification process for certificate holders in the 1990s.

• Concerns about the burden on physicians, relevance and value of periodic recertification multiple-choice examinations, and advances in the science of adult learning have led the ABMS to pursue longitudinal assessment platforms that are seen as more relevant, efficient, flexible, and user-friendly by physicians.

INTRODUCTION
Definitions

Lifelong learning
The voluntary, self-initiated, and continuous search for new knowledge for professional or personal reasons.

Continuing professional development
A process of lifelong learning that begins during graduate medical education and continues for the length of the professional's career. Continuing professional development (CPD) is a professional's responsibility to monitor and reflect on his/her performance, identify practice gaps, and engage and learn activities to improve practice.

Department of Psychiatry and Behavioral Sciences, Feinberg School of Medicine, Northwestern University, 942 Lathrop Avenue, River Forest, IL 60305, USA
[1] Present address: Department of Psychiatry and Behavioral Sciences, 446 East Ontario, 7th Floor, Chicago, IL 60611.
E-mail address: janzia@nm.org

Psychiatr Clin N Am 44 (2021) 309–316
https://doi.org/10.1016/j.psc.2021.03.001
0193-953X/21/© 2021 Elsevier Inc. All rights reserved.

Abbreviations	
ABMS	American Board of Medical Specialties
ABOG	American Board of Obstetrics and Gynecology
ABPN	American Board of Psychiatry and Neurology
ACGME	Accreditation Council for Graduate Medical Education
CPD	Continuing professional development
MOC	Maintenance of Certification

Board certification
The process by which a graduate from an appropriately accredited (Accreditation Council for Graduate Medical Education [ACGME]) psychiatry residency program is determined to be a competent psychiatrist according to the American Board of Psychiatry and Neurology (ABPN), a Member Board of the American Board of Medical Specialties (ABMS). Board certification is an important milestone in the life of a physician.

Continuing certification
Also known as maintenance of certification or MOC. The process by which an ABPN-Certified psychiatrist engages in and verifies his/her CPD.

Clinical skills examinations
Clinical skills examinations (CSEs) and clinical skills verification examinations, are the formative and summative assessment of psychiatry residents' competence in engaging a psychiatric patient, conducting a psychiatric interview, and presenting the case. The evaluator is an ABPN-Certified faculty member. The examination is conducted in real-time with a patient unknown to the resident.

HISTORY OF BOARD CERTIFICATION IN PSYCHIATRY IN THE UNITED STATES
The Early Years

The early 1900s in the United States marked the beginning of a movement toward growth of specialty medicine; in fact, a significant theme in medicine in the twentieth century was the organization of medical specialties and certifying boards. In 1934, the ABPN was created to define specialty requirements and to establish credentials for the practice of psychiatry and neurology. The American Medical Association, the American Psychiatric Association (established in 1844), and the American Neurological Association sponsored this new Board; the 3 organizations still serve as the nominating professional societies for the Board, along with newer additions, the American Academy of Neurology and the American College of Psychiatrists.[1]

The ABPN joined several other certifying Boards; it was the fifth to be formed after the American Board of Ophthalmology (1917), the American Board of Otolaryngology (1924), the Board of Obstetrics and Gynecology (1930), and the Board of Dermatology and Syphilology (1932). This group of Boards was gathered under an umbrella organization in 1933: The Advisory Board for Medical Specialties, which is now known as the ABMS (or the American Board of Medical Specialties). The ABMS currently has 24 member boards and oversees 40 specialties and 87 subspecialties. It sets standards for these boards and manages any conflicts among them. The ABPN now provides certificates for 15 subspecialties within psychiatry and neurology; some, such as palliative care and sleep medicine, are shared with other specialties.

The ABPN created and administered its first examination in 1935; most physicians then practiced both psychiatry and neurology as a combined specialty. In fact, at that first examination, which included 31 candidates, 9 were certified in both psychiatry and neurology, 10 in psychiatry alone, and 2 in neurology alone. From 1934 until 2007, the examination included a live examination of an actual patient or patients. For several decades, the certification examination in psychiatry consisted of 2 parts: part I was a 1-day knowledge-based multiple-choice examination; if the candidate passed that examination, he or she was eligible to take part II, which consisted of an evaluation of specific clinical skills and clinical reasoning with a live patient or patients; later, videos and then written vignettes of patients were added to the examination of a live patient.

The part II examination evolved, but continued to present numerous challenges and problems, including patient variability, problems with reliability measures, the extraordinary expense and logistics of requiring large numbers of examiners and candidates to travel to one city for the examination. The examination was also a one-time high-stakes examination, which could affect candidates' ability to perform as they routinely would in the workplace. Candidate anxiety was usually very high in the setting of such an expensive examination with such significant career consequences. In 2007, the ABPN leadership decided to discontinue the part II examination and move the evaluation of core skills into the residency training years and included the following: (1) candidates' ability to form an appropriate physician-patient relationship, (2) candidates' ability to conduct a psychiatric interview, and (3) candidates' ability to deliver an organized, accurate and comprehensive presentation of the case.

In collaboration with the ACGME Psychiatry Review Committee, the ABPN established a new in-residency requirement: the successful completion of 3 clinical skills examinations. The "pass" standard was the performance level of a competent psychiatrist practicing in the community. The purpose of the examination is formative and summative; a resident can complete as many CSEs as desired and learn and improve with each effort until able to complete 3 "pass" examinations. Three "passing" CSEs became a requirement for graduation from an ACGME-accredited psychiatry program, as well as a requirement for eligibility to take the Board certification examination following graduation. When CSEs were established, the ACGME, the ABPN, and American Association of Directors of Psychiatry Residency Training, the psychiatry training directors' organization, established evaluator training modules for faculty who would be conducting the examinations. In psychiatry, the last oral board examination was the child and adolescent part II examination in 2016.

Some research has explored reliability measures in CSEs, including 1 multisite study looking at interrater reliability in groups of evaluators from different academic sites. At least 1 multisite research study supports the reliability of the CSEs.

The summative Certification Examination, which is now a full-day multiple-choice examination administered through a national testing organization, is created in a multiple-step process; questions undergo many iterations and edits that the ABPN then pilots before adding them to the examination. The ABPN has instituted a 2-dimensional topic format for all multiple-choice examinations, one axis for diagnoses and the second axis for competency areas (diagnosis, patient care, professionalism, for example). Test assembly ensures that there is an adequate number of questions in each diagnostic and competency area. There has been an increased focus on creating test questions that include clinical vignettes followed by a series of questions focused on clinical reasoning and context. The ABPN has created new video clinical vignettes using professional actors and scripts based on actual clinical encounters written by ABPN Committees. Psychometrics of each examination are reviewed continually, and examination questions are adjusted accordingly.

Changes in Expectations: Continuing Professional Development

Starting in the 1990s and increasing in the early 2000s, input from various governmental agencies, institutions, and advocacy organizations generated a mandate for ensuring that physicians maintained and improved their knowledge and skills over time: lifelong learning for physicians. Research in the neuroscience of human learning challenged previous pedagogical methods in continuing medical education. This research demonstrated that passive learning through mass reading followed by lengthy high-stakes examinations (the typical method used by Member Boards of the ABMS) was an ineffective learning method for retaining knowledge and skills. There was accumulating evidence that many patients in the United States were not receiving evidence-based care, which led to stakeholder demands for greater physician accountability, a better quality of care, and patient safety. Factors such as global demographics, constant access to new information, and the need for rapid dissemination of scientific advances heighten the importance of continuous lifelong learning.[2]

After 60 years of giving lifetime board certificates for psychiatry, in the early 1990s, the ABMS mandated that Member Boards initiate 10-year time-limited certificates in all specialties to assure the public that physicians were maintaining their knowledge and skills. Diplomates who had received lifetime certificates were able to maintain them. The ABPN then began creating recertification examinations for the 2 specialties and the subspecialties; these examinations are currently 1-day computer-delivered multiple-choice question examinations administered by a national testing center. Diplomates who were certified after 1994 must take the examination every 10 years after their initial Board Certification.

In 2014, the ABMS created new standards for their program of MOC.[3] The standards required that each Member Board incorporate all ACGME/ABMS core competencies in its program, work to "increase the Program's quality, relevance, and meaningfulness," and engage in continuous quality monitoring and improvement of the MOC programs. The standards also required that each Member Board "identify professionalism expectations for all diplomates." The ABMS stressed that Member Boards must establish lifelong self-assessment and learning requirements, such as tools to identify practice gaps and learning new advances. The outline for the ABPN approach to Continuing Certification is based on the ABMS 2015 Standards and has the 4 following parts:

Part I: Professional standing
Part II: Lifelong learning (continuing medical education and self-assessment)
Part III: Summative assessment of knowledge, judgment, and skills (the 10-year multiple-choice examination)
Part IV: Improvement in medical practice

Some ABMS Member Boards created alternatives to the end-of-cycle examinations early in the initial years of MOC requirements. For example, the American Board of Anesthesiology launched a pilot program called "MOCA Minute" in 2014; this is an interactive learning tool that sends knowledge and skills questions to diplomates regularly and provides immediate feedback on performance. The ABMS gave final approval to this pilot in 2018. For many years, the American Board of Obstetrics and Gynecology (ABOG) delivered article-reading assignments from peer-reviewed literature on clinically relevant topics, treatment guidelines, and essential research. Every year, ABOG presents approximately 150 articles to diplomates in 50 article groups; over the year, diplomates must choose 30 of the 150 articles, read them, and answer 4 assessment questions about the articles. Diplomates must score 80% on the questions in order to retain certification. At the end of year 6 of each MOC cycle, diplomates also must pass a secure computer-based examination at a testing center. In 2019, the ABMS approved a program in which ABOG diplomates who score 86% or higher on the article-based assessments could opt out of the one-time computer-based 6-year examination; this program is called the Performance Pathway.

During and after the ABMS introduction of the new standards for MOC, there has been considerable controversy over MOC requirements, with varying intensity among specialties. Even if there was no negative attitude toward continuing certification and the ABMS and Member Boards, physicians are concerned about the time required, personal costs, burnout, work/life balance issues, and the absence of clear CME goals. Some groups have been concerned about possible conflicts of interest within the Specialty Boards. Also, there is some misinformation among diplomates about the role of ABMS relative to licensing bodies and hospital accreditation organizations—although the ABMS does not influence these groups, and licensure does not require board certification, some physicians questioned whether there was a genuine firewall between the organizations.

Recent Developments: The American Board of Psychiatry and Neurology Pilot Program

In 2018, the ABPN launched a Pilot Program in MOC to offer an alternative to the high-stakes, 10-year examination. The program's goals are to offer more convenient, relevant, and flexible learning and self-assessment for diplomates than the 10-year examination. Also, the program allows choosing articles that psychiatrists judge to be most intriguing and relevant to them from an extensive selection of options. It allows the diplomate the opportunity to complete the reading and assessments at personally convenient times, at any location where Internet access is available. The Pilot Program alternative is an online article-based examination that diplomates can take over 3 years; diplomates who enroll in the program choose 30 out of an available 40 possible journal articles in 10 different diagnostic areas, and after reading each article will take a brief, 5-question online test about the article. The diplomates can take as much time as they wish to answer the questions and must answer at least 4 out of 5 questions to pass the mini-quiz. Diplomates receive the mini-test results immediately after they complete each quiz, and they can also give feedback about the articles, the questions, and their overall examination experience. Also, diplomates could question the correctness of quiz answers; in response, the examination committee would again review the question in light of the feedback and make any necessary corrections in real-time. The flexible time format and the relatively short, current articles and short quizzes focused on the clinical use of relevant knowledge are all advances that align with best practices in adult learning.

Three groups of diplomates were eligible for the Pilot Program: those completing their MOC cycles in 2019, 2020, and 2021. The first group was required to complete 30 articles in 1 year; the second group was required to complete 30 articles in 2 years; and the third group was required to complete 30 articles in 3 years. As of January 2021, 10,052 out of 14,615 eligible diplomates, 69%, registered for the Pilot Program in Adult Psychiatry. Of those, 41% completed all 30 articles and assessments successfully. In the Child and Adolescent Psychiatry Pilot Program, 2316 out of 3311 eligible diplomates, 70%, had registered, and 31% had completed all 30 articles and assessments successfully. The Pilot Program's diplomate satisfaction, judged from the post-quiz questionnaires, is much higher than average satisfaction ratings for the standard ABPN examinations. The ABMS approved (ABPN, personal communication, 2021) the Pilot in the fall of 2020, and it will soon become a standard option for all diplomates.

Recent Developments: American Board of Psychiatry and Neurology "Achieving the Vision for Continuing Board Certification"

In 2018, the ABMS created a new initiative for continuing certification. The "Vision" process convened multiple stakeholders to create a continuing board certification system that is "meaningful, relevant, and of value to physicians." One of the core components of this statement recommends "agreement of all 24 ABMS Member Boards to commit to longitudinal or other formative assessment strategies and offer alternatives to the highly secure, point-in-time examinations of knowledge."[4] Most Specialty Boards have already developed longitudinal assessment programs or are in the process of doing so. Also, the initiative requires that the ABMS develop "new, integrated standards for continuing certification programs by 2020." The ABMS then created 4 collaborative task forces, including one on professionalism. The ABMS will post the proposed recommendations for stakeholder comments in April 2021.

Medicine, including psychiatry, faces numerous future challenges as stakeholders in medical education attempt to develop new methods of ensuring current physician competency and professional development while avoiding undue burden on physicians. The ideal program will be one in which physicians will receive current updated scientific information, assess their knowledge and skills using an external assessment instrument, and develop and pursue learning plans in a flexible and very feasible format. The ideal CPD not only would promote professional growth in knowledge and skills but also would improve physician well-being and patient care. Some Specialty Boards (including the APBN) have discussed using technologies such as avatars and artificial intelligence as potential tools for physicians to assess clinical skills, and future technologies may enable more sophisticated programs that use better techniques for adult learning.

BOARD CERTIFICATION, CONTINUING CERTIFICATION, AND ALIGNMENT WITH CONTINUING PROFESSIONAL DEVELOPMENT

The goals of Board Certification, Continuing Certification, and CPD are overlapping but different. The purpose of the first 2 goals is (1) to protect the public and (2) for diplomates to demonstrate to colleagues, patients, and health care organizations that they meet a standard of competence in the specialty. CPD has a broader purpose for the individual physician, grounded in the commitment to oneself and one's patients: the wish to do well by one's patients and deliver the best possible care. Hilty and colleagues[5] describe CPD as part of physicians' overall well-being, along with self-care elements. The investigators describe a range of CPD activities, such as reflection, directed reading, peer consultation, case conferences, and self- and peer assessment, all performed over a professional lifetime.

One of the Most Common Complaints About the Maintenance of Certification/Continuing Certification

One of the most common complaints about the MOC/Continuing Certification processes in psychiatry is there is a dearth of evidence that participation improves clinician practice and clinical outcomes. Correlating lifelong learning activities and improvement in clinical outcomes is very challenging. Some of the educational activities from medical school didactics through programs offered by professional societies do not use pretests and posttests or assessment tools that can document learning from the activity; more often, there is a subjective report from the learner about how they will change their practice as a result, or asking if the learner was satisfied with the activity. However, some CPD activities have demonstrated improvement in physicians' clinical competence and improved physician performance. In their study, Cerveros and Gaines[6] found that the forms of continuing education most likely to impact both of these factors included using multiple modalities and methods. Some of the most effective methods used spaced exposures that were interactive, longitudinal, and focused on retrieval and outcomes. These methods constitute many of the same principles of effective adult learning described by Brown's survey of educational methods, *Make It Stick.*[7]

Descriptions of CPD describe self-assessment as an essential part of identifying gaps in knowledge and skills. However, there is abundant evidence that physicians' self-assessments of competency are biased and do not correlate well with external ratings. Davis and colleagues[8] demonstrated that physicians with the lowest external assessments were the most likely to overestimate their competency. This alarming finding is one reason external assessments, such as the part III section of the ABMS Continuing Certification process, are crucial to physicians' CPD plans and essential to assure the public that physicians have kept up-to-date in knowledge and skills. Professional societies offer many self-assessment tools in psychiatry, such as the American Psychiatric Association and the American College of Psychiatrists. The ABPN offers some self-assessment credit for the completed Pilot MOC Program and lists many approved assessment tools on the organization Web site that diplomates can use to meet the self-assessment requirement required for Continuing Certification.

The Federation of State Medical Boards and The National Board of Medical Examiners created the Postlicensure Assessment System. Its initial purpose was to assess physicians whose competence was in question, but it is also useful for physicians who wish to assess their medical knowledge, clinical judgment, and patient management skills.

DISCUSSION

The coming decade in US medical education promises to be one of considerable change and innovation; in particular, there will be challenges in ensuring that psychiatrists and other physicians regularly master new knowledge and skills while balancing ever-busier responsibilities in health care. Finding ways to overcome the stigma surrounding Continuing Certification will be necessary, as will the development of educational tools that can demonstrably improve physician competence and patient outcomes. Efforts to align the Continuing Certification process with the core values and methods of CPD, including discoveries in the science of adult learning and new technologies, will be crucial for creating an effective program that both physicians and patients can welcome.

CLINICS CARE POINT

- Although seen as an extra burden, well-developed lifelong learning methods now exist that can function as an essential part of a psychiatrist's professional development.
- The most effective strategies for adult learning should be a part of continuing professional development: programs should be longitudinal, interactive, have interleaving of topics, and present opportunities for memory retrieval.

DISCLOSURE

The author is a current Director of the American Board of Psychiatry and Neurology.

REFERENCES

1. Scheiber SC, Madaan V, Wilson DR. The American Board of Psychiatry and Neurology: historical overview and current perspectives. Psychiatr Clin North Am 2008 Mar;31(1):123–35.
2. Kalz M. Lifelong learning and its support with new technologies. In: Smelser NJ, Baltes PB, editors. International Encyclopedia of the Social and Behavioral Sciences. Pergamon: Oxford; 2015.
3. Standards for the ABMS Program for Maintenance of Certification (MOC) 2014. Available at: abms.org/media/1109/standards-for-the-abms-program-for-moc-fimal.pdf. Accessed January 15, 2014.
4. Available at: https://www.abms.org/news-events/abms-board-of-directors-announces-plan-to-implement-recommendations-from-the-continuing-board-certification-vision-commission-final-report/. Accessed March 19, 2019.
5. Drude KP, Maheu M, Hilty DM. Continuing Professional Development: Reflections on Lifelong Learning Process. Psychiatr Clin North Am 2019 Sep;42(3):447-61.
6. Cervero RM, Gaines JK. The impact of CME on physician performance and patient health outcomes: an updated synthesis of systematic reviews. J Contin Educ Health Prof 2015;35(2):131–8.
7. Brown PC. Make it Stick: the science of successful learning. Cambridge, Massachusetts: The Belknap Press of Harvard University Press; 2014.
8. Davis DA, Mazmanian PE, Fordis M, et al. Accuracy of physician self-assessment compared with observed measures of competence: a systematic review. JAMA 2006;296(9):1094–102.

Advancing Workplace-Based Assessment in Psychiatric Education

Key Design and Implementation Issues

John Q. Young, MD, MPP, PhD[a],*, Jason R. Frank, MD, MA(Ed), FRCPC[b],
Eric S. Holmboe, MD[c]

KEYWORDS

- Workplace-based assessment • Competency-based assessment
- Medical education • Psychiatry • Feedback • Validity
- Entrustable professional activities • Programmatic assessment

KEY POINTS

- Reforms in medical education have led to the adoption of competency frameworks and a reorienting of the curriculum toward these newly defined competencies.
- The focus of assessment has shifted from knows and knows how to what the trainee does with patients and team members in the workplace.
- This shift in the focus of assessment has led to the development of workplace-based assessment.
- Workplace-based assessment programs typically have 2 foci: assessment for learning (formative) and assessment of learning (summative).
- High-quality workplace-based assessment programs require thoughtful choices about the framework of assessment, the tools themselves, the platforms used, and the contexts in which the assessments take place, with an emphasis on direct observation.

Funding: J.Q. Young – ABPN Research Award (2019–2020).
[a] Department of Psychiatry, Donald and Barbara Zucker School of Medicine at Hofstra/Northwell and, Zucker Hillside Hospital at Northwell Health, 75-59 263rd Street, Kaufman Building, Glen Oaks, NY 11004, USA; [b] Department of Emergency Medicine, University of Ottawa, Royal College of Physicians and Surgeons of Canada, 774 Echo Drive, Ottawa, Ontario K15 5NB, Canada; [c] Accreditation Council for Graduate Medical Education, ACGME, 401 North Michigan Avenue, Chicago, IL 60611, USA
* Corresponding author.
E-mail address: Jyoung9@northwell.edu

Abbreviations	
ACGME	Accreditation Council for Graduate Medical Education
CBA	Competency-based assessment
EPAs	Entrustable professional activities
P-SCO	Psychopharmacotherapy-Structured Clinical Observation
PsyME	Psychiatric medical education
WBA	Workplace-based assessment

BACKGROUND
Origins of Competency-Based Medical Education

Over the past 2 plus decades, numerous national and international reports have found critical deficiencies in medical education, including psychiatric medical education (PsyME). These deficiencies include suboptimal patient outcomes, unacceptable variability in the abilities of trainees upon graduation, poor alignment between what trainees learn and the competencies required to provide safe and effective care in twenty-first century health care systems, and a significant gap between evidence-based instructional technique and actual practice in medical education.[1–4] These and other reports have called for fundamental and far-reaching reforms.[5,6]

In response, regulatory bodies transitioned from solely emphasizing structure and process measures (eg, time-based rotations) to including educational outcomes.[7–9] Competency-based medical education, including competency-based assessment (CBA), emerged as an approach to designing and implementing outcomes-based education in medicine.[9] The fundamental premise of competency-based medical education is that trainees should acquire the abilities necessary to meet the health needs of our patients and communities. The competencies are, therefore, derived from an analysis of what a physician must be able to perform in the emerging care delivery models. Competencies, derived in this way, should guide curricula and assessments.[10]

Indeed, many promising innovations have occurred both with respect to content (what is learned) and pedagogy (how the learning occurs). Based on the tasks and roles that physicians must currently perform, the core competencies now include interpersonal communication (eg, interprofessional teamwork), system-based practice (eg, patient safety and quality improvement, health care disparities, social determinants of health), and practice-based learning and improvement (eg, evidence-based medicine).[1,2] The primary curricular focus has evolved from individual-based, episodic management of acute illness to team-based, population-oriented, and technology-enabled longitudinal management of chronic illness.[11] This new focus includes health system sciences as the third pillar that complements the biomedical and clinical sciences.[12] In addition, reforms have also extended to pedagogy with the adoption of evidence-based instructional techniques that are more learner-centered, interactive, and experiential.[13]

Emergence of Workplace-Based Assessment

However, newly defined competencies required newly developed methods of assessment. In medical education, assessment is the measurement (or gathering of information) of how a trainee performs on a given task (eg, multiple choice question examination) to make inferences about their competence (eg, medical knowledge about psychiatric illness). Traditionally, the focus of assessment in medical education has been on the classroom domains of knows and knows how and more recently shows how. Multiple choice examinations and, then, simulation and objective structured clinical examinations dominated. In the competency-based era of outcomes-based education, the focus of assessment has shifted to the workplace domain of doing, that is, what the trainee actually does in practice. This led to a new approach to assessment called workplace-based assessment (WBA). WBA typically has 2 purposes; the assessment of learning (ie, summative) and the assessment for learning (ie, formative).[14–16] Compared with traditional assessment, which privileged summative assessment, WBA rebalances assessment to include formative assessment as a coequal branch of assessment. WBA has introduced new tools such as multisource feedback and direct observation and feedback. And to help make competencies less abstract, the Accreditation Council for Graduate Medical Education (ACGME) added a developmental dimension to the competency framework. Each of the 6 competency domains were divided into specialty-specific subcompetencies. Then, for each subcompetency, the ACGME crafted a series of milestones, a logical progression of behaviors achieved over time as the learner progresses toward and beyond the threshold for unsupervised practice. Beginning in 2013, the Next Accreditation System required program directors to report biannually on each resident's progress with regard to every milestone.[10]

Despite its strategic importance to CBA, WBA programs have encountered significant challenges. Supervisors and trainees often are inadequately trained in assessment, do not understand the purpose, and interact in settings with insufficient time for WBA activities such as direct observation and/or feedback.[17,18] As a result, faculty and residents report a negative view of WBA programs. They describe their experience of WBA programs as tick box or jumping through the hoops exercises that add stress to already compressed schedules and intrude upon the residents' autonomy.[17,19] These findings are consistent and concerning. Researchers, leaders, and practitioners in PsyME will need to develop strategies that overcome these challenges and more effectively engage faculty and residents in WBA. Otherwise, the primary goals of supporting both formative and summative assessment will not be realized and the viability of competency-based medical education will be threatened. This article reviews promising directions in WBA.

WORKPLACE-BASED ASSESSMENT IN CONTEXT

WBA programs should be designed and developed within a broader system of CBA. This system must simultaneously optimize 3 goals: (1) maximal learning through formative assessment (assessment for learning); (2) robust high-stakes decision-making (eg, promotion or selection) through summative assessment (assessment of learning); and (3) ongoing improvements in the curriculum through programmatic assessment.[20] As such, the CBA system must promote both self-regulated growth and clinical competence as judged by a trustworthy process. The key to effectively doing so is situating WBA within a carefully designed system that has several interacting components: WBA, ongoing faculty development, learning analytics, longitudinal coaching, and trustworthy decision-making processes. The companion article on CBA in psychiatric education details each component of a system of CBA. The remainder of this article explores WBA in detail.

WORKPLACE-BASED ASSESSMENT IN PSYCHIATRIC MEDICAL EDUCATION

WBAs focus on what trainees actually do with patients and team members. What the trainee does becomes the basis for identifying growth edges and determining readiness for advancement and, ultimately, independent practice. Implementing WBAs requires choices about the assessment framework, type and design of tool, platforms, rater variability, and the contexts in which assessment will occur.

Framework for Assessment

In developing the WBAs, postgraduate medical education programs must first choose the framework for assessment. The 2 most common developmental frameworks for operationalizing competency-based medical education are milestones and entrustable professional activities (EPAs) (**Fig. 1**). Milestones are more granular. Milestones are behavioral narratives that mark the developmental progression of a trainee's abilities (knowledge, skills, and attitudes) within a given subcompetency. Milestones give definition to the more abstract competencies and, when taken together, milestones depict a model for a trainee's abilities at each stage of development from novice to expert. In contrast, EPAs are more holistic. EPAs are the list of tasks that define a specialty (eg, performing a diagnostic psychiatric assessment).[21] EPAs must be executable within a given time frame, observable, measurable, and suitable for focused entrustment decisions; that is, the task can be entrusted to the trainee for unsupervised execution once sufficient competence is reached.[22] EPAs and milestones are complementary. In other words, an individual requires abilities to perform an activity effectively. EPAs can be mapped to subcompetencies and milestones. Guides have been developed to help groups develop EPAs.[22] Both Canada and the Netherlands have combined milestones and EPAs in their national WBA programs.[23]

The ACGME will implement version 2.0 of the psychiatry milestones in July 2021. Although the ACGME has not adopted EPAs, many specialties have. EPAs have been developed for most specialties, including anesthesiology, ambulatory practice family medicine, gastroenterology, geriatric medicine, hematology and oncology, internal medicine, pediatrics, obstetrics and gynecology, psychiatry, pulmonary and critical care, and rheumatology.[22,24–29] Several different types of expert consensus methodologies have been used, including task forces, interview, and survey. In psychiatry, EPAs were first developed in New Zealand and Australia.[30] Later, a single US residency program implemented EPA-based end-rotation evaluations. In this study, the EPAs were constructed by the rotation leaders.[28]

Recognizing the potential for end-of-training EPAs in the United States, the Executive Council of the American Association of Directors of Psychiatry Residency Training created the EPAs for the Psychiatry Task Force in 2014. The council charged the task force to develop proposed EPAs that every graduating resident should be able to perform without supervision. The task force used a rigorous, multistage process that culminated in a national Delphi survey to develop EPAs that were essential, clear, and representative. This process, the most comprehensive to date for psychiatry, yielded 13 EPAs.[31]

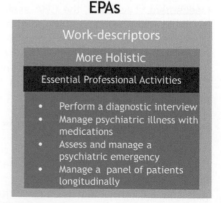

Fig. 1. The rubric of a single response multiple-choice question.

The study authors encouraged programs to experiment and adapt the EPAs to align with local context and mission. For example, programs may choose to lump or split EPAs in various ways:

- Disease (eg, manage bipolar illness versus manage psychiatric disorders)
- Setting (eg, diagnostic psychiatric interview in any setting versus the emergency department)
- Treatment modality (eg, initiate treatment with medications versus clozapine or provide psychotherapy versus provide cognitive behavioral therapy)
- Patient acuity and complexity (eg, patients with one defined problem vs patients with multiple problems).

The American Association of Directors of Psychiatry Residency Training EPA Task Force also recommended differentiating between EPAs that should be required nationally versus those that might be required only by a specific institution and between EPAs that are required, elective, and/or aspirational. Some psychiatry programs have implemented EPAs,[28,32] and the Assessment Committee for the American Association of Directors of Psychiatry Residency Training has published an implementation toolkit for program directors.[33]

Workplace-based assessment fit for purpose

Because assessment drives learning, it is critical that PsyME programs align their WBA tools with their curriculum.[34] This has several implications. Programs must design their WBAs so that each primary EPA or competency is assessed multiple times by several methods. In addition, programs should emphasize a given WBA tool in proportion to the importance of the competencies or EPA that it assesses. The WBAs should indicate to the learner what the program values. Too often, programs assess what is easy to assess rather than what is important. This practice can lead stakeholders to experience WBAs as trivial and intrusive and, worse yet, lead them to focus their learning efforts on relatively less important competencies.

Each WBA tool should possess the key elements of fit-for-purpose individual assessments, with priority given to the validity, feasibility, educational, and catalytic effects, as well as acceptability (**Table 1**).[35-38] The distinction between educational and

Table 1	
Key elements of assessments fit for purpose	
Element	**Description**
Validity	A body of evidence that supports the use of the results of the WBA for the intended purpose. This usually includes evidence related content, internal structure, response process, association with other variables, and consequences.
Feasibility	Implementation of the WBA is doable given the circumstances and context.
Educational effect	Anticipation of the WBA prompts the learners to engage in preparatory activities that have educational benefit.
Catalytic effect	Feedback from the WBA promotes growth and motivates effort and engagement.
Acceptability	The stakeholders, including learners, faculty, clinical competency committees, institutions, and external regulators view the information derived from the WBAs as credible.

Data from: Norcini J, Anderson B, Bollela V, et al. Criteria for good assessment: consensus statement and recommendations from the Ottawa 2010 Conference. *Med Teach.* 2011;33(3):206-214.

catalytic effects is important. Educational effects refer to the effects on behavior that occur before the WBA, that is, to what extent anticipation of the WBA prompts the learner to engage in preparatory activities that are valuable and worth the time. Catalytic effects refer to the effects of the WBA after the assessment, that is, to what extent does the WBA generate information and feedback that prompts both growth and future motivated effort. WBAs should motivate high-yield activities both before and after the assessment.

PsyME programs should use multiple types of WBAs, each administered multiple times with multiple assessors.[20] The use of multiples helps to overcome important sources of bias. Multiple methods help to compensate for the limitations of any single technique. Multiple assessments of a given competency or EPA help to overcome one-offs (eg, resident performing atypically) and to develop a more stable and complete view of a trainee's skill. Multiple assessors compensates for the biases (eg, halo effects, leniency, race, gender, etc...) that influence any given faculty member's judgment.

Workplace-Based Assessment: Types of Tools

The most common WBA tools include multisource feedback (patients, staff, and peers), chart stimulated recall, direct observation, end-rotation global feedback, portfolios, and practice-based audits (Table 2). Multisource feedback tools typically focus on the competency domains of interpersonal communication and professionalism from the perspective of faculty, allied health staff, patients, peers, administrative staff, and the self. Several studies have shown that psychiatry residents value this feedback.[39–41] Chart stimulated recall has not been studied in psychiatry, but represents an excellent way to assess clinical reasoning and decision-making. For example, an attending may view the chart of a patient recently seen by the resident and then ask for the rationale behind the clinical decisions and probe further by asking a series of hypothetical "what ifs" (eg, what if the patient was pregnant, would your choice of medication change? How would you explain the risk of medication y to such a patient?).[42]

The Psychopharmacotherapy-Structured Clinical Observation (P-SCO) is the direct observation and feedback tool in psychiatry with the most evidence for validity. The P-SCO was developed to assess the EPA of a follow-up (medication management) visit.[43] The P-SCO includes a checklist of the essential tasks of a medication visit plus space for narrative comments. The feasibility and usefulness of implementing the P-SCO has been demonstrated in several studies.[43,44] Additional research has reported evidence for the validity of the P-SCO with respect to its content, internal structure, and association with other variables.[45,46] Moreover, the P-SCO has been found to generate high-quality narrative comments that are behaviorally specific and balanced between corrective and reenforcing and either add unique content or elaborate on the why behind a low or high quantitative score.[43,47] This latter finding is particularly encouraging, given that research on end-rotation evaluations has found narrative comments to be vague and nonspecific and, therefore, ineffective.[43,48] Evidence for validity has also been developed for the EPA of a psychiatric diagnostic interview.[49] Finally, a mobile app that assesses EPAs in psychiatry showed evidence of feasibility and validity.[50] The completion of a single assessment with the EPA app took on average 72 seconds and generated 1 high-quality, specific, corrective comment. The entrustment scores assigned by faculty using the EPA app correlated highly with the experience level of the trainee.

Although the use of portfolios as a WBA tool has been demonstrated in psychiatry, relatively little has been written.[51,52] Finally, perhaps the most underused WBA method in psychiatry is practice-based audit or the provision of meaningful outcomes

Table 2
Common examples of workplace-based assessment approaches

Approach	Description	Example
Multisource feedback	Assessments from patients, staff, and peers, typically focused on interpersonal communication and professionalism.	Patient experience surveys in which the results can be tied to a specific trainee.
Direct observation and structured feedback	Assessments from supervisors based on the direct observation of the trainee performing a clinical task.	Psychopharmacotherapy – Structured Clinical Observation Tool
Chart stimulated recall	Assessment based on a trainee's responses to a series of "what if" questions based on an actual patient (ie, chart).	To assess competence with managing depression in peripartum patients, each resident answers questions such as how would their approach to the management of depression change if they learned that the patient has a history of a manic episode.
Practice-based audit	Assessment based on measures for meaningful outcomes that derive from the clinical care the trainee delivered to patients.	A quarterly dashboard that shows for each trainee what proportion of their patients on antipsychotic medications have received appropriate metabolic screening.
Portfolio	Assessment based on a systematic collection and organization of artifacts that represent the ability to perform a task. Portfolios often include a reflective component.	Trainees post on a digital platform copies of several biopsychosocial formulations they wrote or videos of teaching a patient how to do an exposure exercise with reflections.

(eg, proportion of patients on an antipsychotic medication who have been screen for the metabolic syndrome according to guidelines) derived from the clinical care delivered by the learner to their patients. Groundbreaking work in pediatrics has identified resident-sensitive quality measures, that is, measures influenced by the care delivered by residents and obtainable from electronic records.[53–55] Similar efforts are urgently needed in PsyME.

Future research in PsyME should focus on the development of WBAs that focus on EPAs and competencies other than the relatively well-studied follow-up visit and diagnostic interview. Priority areas include WBAs for psychotherapies, quality improvement and patient safety, clinical reasoning, handoffs, and critical appraisal and evidence-based medicine. To meet this need, PsyME educators and researchers can either develop new tools or adapt those with evidence for validity in other specialties.[56–58]

Workplace-Based Assessment: Design

Regardless, WBAs should include both quantitative and, importantly, narrative data.[59–62] A recent study of the P-SCO found that the checklist and the narrative comments complemented each other. The narrative comments amplified on the low or high checklist scores, providing important explanation and guidance to the resident and the clinical competency committee about what was done well or not so well. At the same time, one-half of the comments addressed aspects of the performance not captured by the checklist, contributing highly valuable content that otherwise would not be captured.[47] Some programs are using WBAs with only comments. The rationale is that completing the checklist or quantitative items comes at a cost, both in terms of time and rater cognitive load.[63] In addition, some studies suggest that learners find the comments more helpful than the quantitative scores, and recent studies suggested that narrative comments can support summative judgments.[59,61,64] On the other hand, the checklist may improve clinical care and feedback by orienting both the supervisor and learner to a shared mental model of what competence looks like in that particular setting. The checklist may also help faculty to identify and provide behaviorally specific feedback. A recent implementation study of the P-SCO supported these benefits.[44] In addition, the completion of the checklist may lead to improvements in the raters' (faculty) own practice.[34] If the frame of reference provided by the checklist does result in higher quality comments, then several important questions must be answered. Is provision of the checklist (rather than completion) adequate, or is completion necessary in order to generate high quality and reliable comments? If completion is essential, is there a threshold number of completed observations after which the checklist is sufficiently internalized by the faculty member and no longer necessary? And does the checklist help the learner progress more rapidly? As we look to the sustainability of our direct observation assessment programs, these questions will be important to answer through future research on the P-SCO and other direct observation tools.

Workplace-Based Assessment Platforms

The CBA system must also choose carefully the platforms for its WBAs. The principal choices are paper based versus mobile apps. Research in PsyME has identified trade-offs. A series of studies using implementation science to identify the barriers and facilitators of engagement with both an EPA app and a paper-based WBA yielded several insights.[44,65] First, it is critical that mobile apps be developed using an iterative, user-centered process to minimize cognitive load and ensure ease of use (feasibility) and high quality data.[63,66–68] User-centered design processes leverage focus groups, think-alouds, and human factors principles to iteratively design, test, and redesign the tool. This process is relevant to paper-based forms as well. Well-designed, easy-to-use tools are much more likely to be used in the manner intended. Second, careful attention should be given to how WBAs, whether electronic or paper, are embedded within clinical workflows to ensure feasibility.[37] Alpha and beta testing can help to identify features of the WBA and/or workflow that either facilitate or impede engagement such as how many, when, and for how long patients are scheduled. Third, these studies found that faculty and residents value the quickness of the mobile app and how the app forced the faculty member to distill feedback into a succinct point. In contrast, both faculty and residents appreciated how the paper-based form with a checklist generated more thorough, systematic feedback. Faculty, however, stated that they would resent completing the checklist on a smartphone. These studies suggests that there is a role for both types of platforms (and tools) in a WBA program.

Variance: Friend or Foe?

Variance will exist. The traditional psychometric approach to assessment aims to decrease as much as possible inter-rater variability. In the context of WBAs that assess complex competencies, it is important to differentiate between variability that is unwarranted versus variability that arises from assessors perceiving or inferring or focusing on equally valid, but different, dimensions of performance.[69] Two faculty may rate the same resident encounter with a patient differently. These differences can arise for multiple reasons. Each faculty may value 2 different, equally important components of the task. One attending may focus their comments on the systematic use of criteria-based questions for diagnosis, whereas another may focus their feedback on the use of verbal and nonverbal techniques to enhance the therapeutic alliance and the validity of the patient's answers to the diagnostic questions. In this case, both faculty, although perhaps overly focused on their particular favorite theme, are correct. The variance in this case that arises from multiple assessors enhances the quality of the feedback. This is good variance. In contrast, 1 faculty may not ever evaluate a resident on certain aspects of the task, such as screening for substance misuse. This kind of variance may reflect contradictory notions of the task and be unwarranted. Thus, although some of the variance will be meaningful and important to embrace, some will also arise from bias or incorrect conceptions of competence (eg, selective abstraction, gender, race, premature judgment, idiosyncratic beliefs, etc). The use of multiple assessments and multiple diverse assessors combined with vigorous performance dimension training can help a WBA program to manage and reduce these tensions.

Direct Observation and Structured Feedback

All WBA programs should include direct observation and structured feedback programs. Such programs facilitate the capture of data at the point of care that can be aggregated into powerful performance dashboards as well as opportunities for coaching in the moment. The implementation of direct observation and structured feedback programs have encountered significant challenges. Supervisors and trainees often are trained inadequately, do not understand the purpose, and interact in settings with insufficient time for direct observation and/or feedback.[17,18] Studies have identified additional barriers such as brief and frequently changing supervisory relationships that do not permit the development of strong educational alliances and low-quality, unidirectional feedback that is not credible to the trainee.[70–77] Moreover, trainees often perceive assessment as summative, even when intended as formative.[78–80] Trainees may alter their behavior (eg, adopt a checklist approach) to conform to what they perceive to be desired.[19,81] The direct observation then morphs into a performance that feels inauthentic and, in turn, undermines subsequent receptivity to feedback (eg, "that is not what I normally do anyways").[19] As a result, some studies indicate that faculty and residents have a negative view of direct observation and structured feedback programs. They describe their experience as tick the box or jumping through the hoops exercises that add stress to already compressed schedules and intrude on the residents' autonomy.[17,19]

To address these challenges, researchers have proposed a number of strategies[17,18,71,82,83] (Box 1). Clinic and attending schedules must be modified to create the protected space for observation and structured feedback.[17,18] This practice can lead to decreased clinical productivity. However, some programs have offset many of these costs by billing for observation time as professional services. Robust and deliberate practice with coaching can accelerate skill acquisition and then permit learners to be entrusted with more patient care responsibilities later in training, leading to additional cost mitigation. Other critical strategies for direct observation and structured feedback programs include ongoing faculty and resident training, longitudinal supervisory relationships, the use of feedback models that emphasize bidirectiona, coconstructed conversations, structured WBA tools with evidence for validity as described elsewhere in this article, and monitoring of engagement.

Box 1
Key features of successful direct observation and structured feedback programs

1. Ongoing faculty and resident training
    a. Direct observation, including how to support resident autonomy while observing;
    b. Use of the chosen WBAs, with attention to performance dimensions, frame of reference, and narrative comments;
    c. Engaging in feedback conversation via a 4-step process: establish an alliance and self-assessment, feedback (with an emphasis on open ended higher order questions and facilitated listening), encouragement, and direction.
2. Longitudinal supervisor–trainee relationships
3. Repeated, frequent observations
4. Protected time for faculty observe and for faculty and trainee
5. Feedback practiced as a coconstructed, bidirectional conversation
6. Structured observation tools with evidence for validity
7. Engagement monitored

A recent qualitative study of a direct observation program in psychiatry found that when these strategies are bundled together many of these challenges can be overcome.[84] Faculty and residents were aligned around the goals. They both perceived the program as focused on growth rather than judgment, even though residents understood that the feedback had both formative and summative purposes. The program facilitated educational alliances characterized by trust and respect. With repeated practice within a longitudinal relationship, trainees dropped the performance orientation and described their interactions with patients as authentic. Residents generally perceived the feedback as credible, described feedback quality as high, and valued the 2-way conversation.

Bundling the strategies in **Box 1** together seemed to bring about an important culture change in which the emphasis was on growth. This outcome is very encouraging. However, there was an important note of caution in this study. When receiving feedback with which they did not agree, residents demurred or, at most, would ask a clarifying question, but then internally discounted the feedback. This finding is not new. On the one hand, skepticism and interrogation is okay. We want learners to critically appraise feedback before judging its credibility and whether to incorporate. Some feedback has more to do with 'style' than 'substance' or may even be incorrect. The fact that learners are discounting some feedback is good. On the other hand, this finding is concerning and represents an important threat to WBA and its ability to help learners grow. Some of the feedback discounted likely was correct or, even if a matter of style, still worth exploration. Further research is needed to understand what kind of feedback is being discounted and how that discounting process impacts growth. This raises the importance of longitudinal coaches that help the trainee learn how to self-assess, interpret performance data, and execute change plans.

DISCUSSION

WBA itself represents a profound change in the approach to assessment. The focus shifts from what the trainee knows to what they do. The goal is not just summative, but also formative. Effective WBA programs will have several features. First, WBA programs should assess each important competency and/or EPA with multiple strategies and assessors on multiple occasions. Common WBA strategies include multisource feedback, direct observation and feedback, practice-based outcome data, chart stimulated recall, and portfolios. Programs should use tools with evidence for validity. Second, the tools and their platforms should be designed with priority given to ease of use and benefit for the end users (eg, faculty, trainees, and clinical competency committees). Direct observation is the backbone of any WBA program. Effective direct observation and structured feedback programs requires bundling together multiple strategies, such as protected faculty time for observation and feedback, longitudinal supervisory relationships, bidirectional feedback models, and ongoing faculty and resident training. The trainings need to develop shared mental models around the performance dimensions, frames of reference, feedback and coaching in the moment, feedback as bidirectional coconstructed conversation, self-regulated learning and change, and how to navigate feedback that one does not agree with or seems to be identity threatening.

In PsyME, several important developments have occurred over the past decade. A rigorous, national Delphi study developed end-of-residency training EPAs and these EPAs have been explicitly linked to the competencies. Evidence for validity has been collected for WBAs for the medication management visit and the diagnostic interview. WBAs have been successfully implemented both on paper and mobile apps. And recent research has identified key enablers of engagement with direct observation and structured feedback.

These developments provide a solid foundation for future efforts. Several important gaps exist. First, EPAs have yet to be developed for fellowships in psychiatry. This needs to be prioritized along with more extensive examination and evaluation of the end-of-residency-training EPAs. Second, PsyME does not have WBAs with validity for evidence for essential competencies and EPAs such as providing (supportive, cognitive-behavioral, and psychodynamic) psychotherapy, managing a psychiatric emergency, sending and receiving a handoff, clinical reasoning, and providing a consultation. Much more work needs to be done in basic WBA tool development. Third, PsyME has not developed models that capture meaningful patient-outcome data linked to individual trainees that can be used for WBA. Finally, WBAs sit within a system of CBA. The WBAs will only be as good as the other components of that system. The WBA must be situated within a carefully designed system that has several interacting components: WBA, ongoing faculty development, learning analytics, longitudinal coaching, and trustworthy decision-making processes. PsyME has much work to do in these other components (eg, learning analytics, dashboards and data visualization, and longitudinal coaching).

In summary, CBA seeks to promote both self-regulated growth and clinical competence as judged by a trustworthy process. To deliver on this promise, programs must have an effective program of WBA. This requires careful choices about the framework of assessment, the tools themselves, the platforms used, and the contexts in which the assessments take place, with an emphasis on direct observation. Much progress has been made in the past decade, which gives us hope about meeting the challenges of the next decade.

DISCLOSURES

The authors have no conflicts of interest to disclose.

REFERENCES

1. Frenk J, Chen L, Bhutta ZA, et al. Health professionals for a new century: transforming education to strengthen health systems in an interdependent world. Lancet 2010;376(9756):1923–58.

2. Lucey CR. Medical education: part of the problem and part of the solution. JAMA Intern Med 2013;173(17):1639–43.
3. Cooke M, Irby DM, O'Brien BC. Carnegie Foundation for the Advancement of Teaching. In: Educating physicians: a call for reform of medical school and residency. 1st edition. San Francisco, CA: Jossey-Bass; 2010.
4. Eden J, Berwick DM, Wilensky GR, Institute of Medicine (U.S), Committee on the Governance and Financing of Graduate Medical Education. Graduate medical education that meets the nation's health needs. Washington, DC: The National Academies Press; 2014.
5. Thibault GE. Reforming health professions education will require culture change and closer ties between classroom and practice. Health Aff (Project Hope) 2013; 32(11):1928–32.
6. Skochelak SE. A decade of reports calling for change in medical education: what do they say? Acad Med 2010;85(9 Suppl):S26–33.
7. Carraccio C, Wolfsthal SD, Englander R, et al. Shifting paradigms: from Flexner to competencies. Acad Med 2002;77(5):361–7.
8. Leach DC. A model for GME: shifting from process to outcomes. A progress report from the Accreditation Council for Graduate Medical Education. Med Educ 2004;38(1):12–4.
9. Frank JR, Snell LS, Cate OT, et al. Competency-based medical education: theory to practice. Med Teach 2010;32(8):638–45.
10. Frank JR, Mungroo R, Ahmad Y, et al. Toward a definition of competency-based education in medicine: a systematic review of published definitions. Med Teach 2010;32(8):631–7.
11. Crosson FJ, Leu J, Roemer BM, et al. Gaps in residency training should be addressed to better prepare doctors for a twenty-first-century delivery system. Health Aff (Project Hope) 2011;30(11):2142–8.
12. Gonzalo JD, Haidet P, Papp KK, et al. Educating for the 21st-century health care system: an interdependent framework of basic, clinical, and systems sciences. Acad Med 2017;92(1):35–9.
13. Irby DM, Cooke M, O'Brien BC. Calls for reform of medical education by the Carnegie Foundation for the advancement of teaching: 1910 and 2010. Acad Med 2010;85(2):220–7.
14. Halman S, Dudek N, Wood T, et al. Direct observation of clinical skills feedback scale: development and validity evidence. Teach Learn Med 2016;28(4):385–94.
15. Miller A, Archer J. Impact of workplace based assessment on doctors' education and performance: a systematic review. BMJ 2010;341:c5064.
16. Schuwirth LW, Van der Vleuten CP. Programmatic assessment: from assessment of learning to assessment for learning. Med Teach 2011;33(6):478–85.
17. Massie J, Ali JM. Workplace-based assessment: a review of user perceptions and strategies to address the identified shortcomings. Adv Health Sci Educ Theor Pract 2016;21(2):455–73.
18. Cheung WJ, Patey AM, Frank JR, et al. Barriers and enablers to direct observation of trainees' clinical performance: a qualitative study using the theoretical domains framework. Acad Med 2019;94(1):101–14.
19. LaDonna KA, Hatala R, Lingard L, et al. Staging a performance: learners' perceptions about direct observation during residency. Med Educ 2017;51(5):498–510.
20. van der Vleuten CP, Schuwirth LW, Driessen EW, et al. A model for programmatic assessment fit for purpose. Med Teach 2012;34(3):205–14.
21. Ten Cate O. Competency-based education, entrustable professional activities, and the power of language. J Grad Med Educ 2013;5(1):6–7.

22. Ten Cate O, Chen HC, Hoff RG, et al. Curriculum development for the workplace using Entrustable Professional Activities (EPAs): AMEE Guide No. 99. Med Teach 2015;37(11):983–1002.
23. Dagnone D, Stockley D, Flynn L, et al. Delivering on the promise of competency based medical education - an institutional approach. Can Med Educ J 2019; 10(1):e28–38.
24. Leipzig RM, Sauvigne K, Granville LJ, et al. What is a geriatrician? American Geriatrics Society and Association of Directors of Geriatric Academic Programs end-of-training entrustable professional activities for geriatric medicine. J Am Geriatr Soc 2014;62(5):924–9.
25. Wisman-Zwarter N, van der Schaaf M, Ten Cate O, et al. Transforming the learning outcomes of anaesthesiology training into entrustable professional activities: a Delphi study. Eur J Anaesthesiol 2016;33(8):559–67.
26. Brown CR Jr, Criscione-Schreiber L, O'Rourke KS, et al. What is a rheumatologist and how do we make one? Arthritis Care Res 2016;68(8):1166–72.
27. Rose S, Fix OK, Shah BJ, et al. Entrustable professional activities for gastroenterology fellowship training. Gastrointest Endosc 2014;80(1):16–27.
28. Weiss A, Ozdoba A, Carroll V, et al. Entrustable professional activities: enhancing meaningful use of evaluations and milestones in a psychiatry residency program. Acad Psychiatry 2016;40(5):850–4.
29. Boyce P, Spratt C, Davies M, et al. Using entrustable professional activities to guide curriculum development in psychiatry training. BMC Med Educ 2011; 11:96.
30. RANZCP. The Royal Australian & New Zealand College of Psychiatrists. EPA Handbook. Available at: https://www.ranzcp.org/Files/PreFellowship/2012-Fellowship-Program/EPA-forms/EPA-handbook.aspx. Accessed January 22, 2017.
31. Young JQ, Hasser C, Hung EK, et al. Developing end-of-training entrustable professional activities for psychiatry: results and methodological lessons. Acad Med 2018;93(7):1048–54.
32. Pinilla S, Lenouvel E, Strik W, et al. Entrustable professional activities in psychiatry: a systematic review. Acad Psychiatry 2020;44(1):37–45.
33. Hung EK, Jibson M, Sadhu J, et al. Wresting with implementation: a step-by-step guide to implementing Entrustable Professional Activities (EPAs) in Psychiatry Residency Programs. Acad Psychiatry 2021;45(2):210–6.
34. Norcini J, Burch V. Workplace-based assessment as an educational tool: AMEE Guide No. 31. Med Teach 2007;29(9):855–71.
35. Downing SM. Validity: on meaningful interpretation of assessment data. Med Educ 2003;37(9):830–7.
36. Lockyer JM, Sargeant J, Richards SH, et al. Multisource feedback and narrative comments: polarity, specificity, actionability, and CanMEDS roles. J Contin Educ Health Prof 2018;38(1):32–40.
37. Norcini J, Anderson MB, Bollela V, et al. 2018 Consensus framework for good assessment. Med Teach 2018;40(11):1102–9.
38. Norcini J, Anderson B, Bollela V, et al. Criteria for good assessment: consensus statement and recommendations from the Ottawa 2010 Conference. Med Teach 2011;33(3):206–14.
39. Grujich NN, Razmy A, Zaretsky A, et al. Evaluation of professional role competency during psychiatry residency. Acad Psychiatry 2012;36(2):126–8.
40. Violato C, Lockyer JM, Fidler H. Assessment of psychiatrists in practice through multisource feedback. Can J Psychiatry 2008;53(8):525–33.

41. Vesel TP, O'Brien BC, Henry DM, et al. Useful but different: resident physician perceptions of interprofessional feedback. Teach Learn Med 2016;28(2):125–34.
42. Philibert I. Using chart review and chart-stimulated recall for resident assessment. J Grad Med Educ 2018;10(1):95–6.
43. Young JQ, Lieu S, O'Sullivan P, et al. Development and initial testing of a structured clinical observation tool to assess pharmacotherapy competence. Acad Psychiatry 2011;35(1):27–34.
44. Young JQ, Sugarman R, Schwartz J, et al. Faculty and resident engagement with a workplace-based assessment tool: use of implementation science to explore enablers and barriers. Acad Med 2020;95(12):1937–44.
45. Young JQ, Irby DM, Kusz M, et al. Performance assessment of pharmacotherapy: results from a content validity survey of the Psychopharmacotherapy-Structured Clinical Observation (P-SCO) Tool. Acad Psychiatry 2018;42(6):765–72.
46. Young JQ, Rasul R, O'Sullivan PS. Evidence for the validity of the psychopharmacotherapy-structured clinical observation tool: results of a factor and time series analysis. Acad Psychiatry 2018;42(6):759–64.
47. Young JQ, Sugarman R, Holmboe E, et al. Advancing our understanding of narrative comments generated by direct observation tools: lessons from the psychopharmacotherapy-structured clinical observation. J Grad Med Educ 2019;11(5):570–9.
48. Ginsburg S, van der Vleuten CP, Eva KW, et al. Cracking the code: residents' interpretations of written assessment comments. Med Educ 2017;51(4):401–10.
49. Jibson MD, Broquet KE, Anzia JM, et al. Clinical skills verification in general psychiatry: recommendations of the ABPN Task Force on Rater Training. Acad Psychiatry 2012;36(5):363–8.
50. Young JQ, McClure M. Fast, easy, and good: assessing entrustable professional activities in psychiatry residents with a mobile app. Acad Med 2020;95(10):1546–9.
51. O'Sullivan PS, Reckase MD, McClain T, et al. Demonstration of portfolios to assess competency of residents. Adv Health Sci Educ Theor Pract 2004;9(4):309–23.
52. Sockalingam S, Stergiopoulos V, Maggi JD, et al. Evaluating psychiatry residents as physician-managers: development of an assessment tool. Acad Psychiatry 2013;37(1):11–7.
53. Schumacher DJ, Holmboe E, Carraccio C, et al. Resident-sensitive quality measures in the pediatric emergency department: exploring relationships with supervisor entrustment and patient acuity and complexity. Acad Med 2020;95(8):1256–64.
54. Schumacher DJ, Holmboe ES, van der Vleuten C, et al. Developing resident-sensitive quality measures: a model from pediatric emergency medicine. Acad Med 2018;93(7):1071–8.
55. Schumacher DJ, Martini A, Holmboe E, et al. Initial implementation of resident-sensitive quality measures in the pediatric emergency department: a wide range of performance. Acad Med 2020;95(8):1248–55.
56. Davis J, Roach C, Elliott C, et al. Feedback and assessment tools for handoffs: a systematic review. J Grad Med Educ 2017;9(1):18–32.
57. ten Cate O, Durning SJ. Approaches to assessing the clinical reasoning of pre-clinical students. In: ten Cate O, Custers E, Durning SJ, editors. Principles and practice of case-based clinical reasoning education: a method for Preclinical Students. Cham, CH: Springer Copyright 2018, The Author(s); 2018. p. 65–72.

58. Cook RJ, Durning SJ. Clinical process modeling: an approach for enhancing the assessment of physicians' clinical reasoning. Acad Med 2019;94(9):1317–22.
59. Ginsburg S, van der Vleuten CPM, Eva KW. The hidden value of narrative comments for assessment: a quantitative reliability analysis of qualitative data. Acad Med 2017;92(11):1617–21.
60. Ginsburg S, Regehr G, Lingard L, et al. Reading between the lines: faculty interpretations of narrative evaluation comments. Med Educ 2015;49(3):296–306.
61. Ginsburg S, Eva K, Regehr G. Do in-training evaluation reports deserve their bad reputations? A study of the reliability and predictive ability of ITER scores and narrative comments. Acad Med 2013;88(10):1539–44.
62. Sargeant J, Armson H, Chesluk B, et al. The processes and dimensions of informed self-assessment: a conceptual model. Acad Med 2010;85(7):1212–20.
63. Tavares W, Ginsburg S, Eva KW. Selecting and simplifying: rater performance and behavior when considering multiple competencies. Teach Learn Med 2016;28(1):41–51.
64. Lefebvre C, Hiestand B, Glass C, et al. Examining the effects of narrative commentary on evaluators' summative assessments of resident performance. Eval Health Prof 2020;43(3):159–61.
65. Young JQ, Sugarman R, Schwartz J, et al. A mobile app to capture EPA assessment data: utilizing the consolidated framework for implementation research to identify enablers and barriers to engagement. Perspect Med Educ 2020;9(4):210–9.
66. Warm EJ, Held JD, Hellmann M, et al. Entrusting observable practice activities and milestones over the 36 months of an internal medicine residency. Acad Med 2016;91(10):1398–405.
67. Saleem JJ, Herout J, Wilck NR. Function-specific design principles for the electronic health record. Proc Hum Factors Ergon Soc Annu Meet 2016;60(1):578–82.
68. Mayer RE, Moreno R. Nine ways to reduce cognitive load in multimedia learning. Educ Psychol 2003;38(1):43–52.
69. Gingerich A, Kogan J, Yeates P, et al. Seeing the 'black box' differently: assessor cognition from three research perspectives. Med Educ 2014;48(11):1055–68.
70. Holmboe E, Ginsburg S, Bernabeo E. The rotational approach to medical education: time to confront our assumptions? Med Educ 2011;45(1):69–80.
71. Ramani S, Konings KD, Ginsburg S, et al. Twelve tips to promote a feedback culture with a growth mind-set: swinging the feedback pendulum from recipes to relationships. Med Teach 2019;41(6):625–31.
72. Ramani S, Post SE, Konings K, et al. "It's just not the culture": a qualitative study exploring residents' perceptions of the impact of institutional culture on feedback. Teach Learn Med 2017;29(2):153–61.
73. Telio S, Ajjawi R, Regehr G. The "educational alliance" as a framework for reconceptualizing feedback in medical education. Acad Med 2015;90(5):609–14.
74. Voyer S, Cuncic C, Butler DL, et al. Investigating conditions for meaningful feedback in the context of an evidence-based feedback programme. Med Educ 2016;50(9):943–54.
75. Sukhera J, Wodzinski M, Milne A, et al. Implicit bias and the feedback paradox: exploring how health professionals engage with feedback while questioning its credibility. Acad Med 2019;94(8):1204–10.
76. Watling C, Driessen E, van der Vleuten CP, et al. Learning from clinical work: the roles of learning cues and credibility judgements. Med Educ 2012;46(2):192–200.

77. Telio S, Regehr G, Ajjawi R. Feedback and the educational alliance: examining credibility judgements and their consequences. Med Educ 2016;50(9):933–42.
78. Bok HG, Teunissen PW, Favier RP, et al. Programmatic assessment of competency-based workplace learning: when theory meets practice. BMC Med Educ 2013;13:123.
79. Harrison C, Wass V. The challenge of changing to an assessment for learning culture. Med Educ 2016;50(7):704–6.
80. Harrison CJ, Konings KD, Schuwirth LWT, et al. Changing the culture of assessment: the dominance of the summative assessment paradigm. BMC Med Educ 2017;17(1):73.
81. Watling C, LaDonna KA, Lingard L, et al. Sometimes the work just needs to be done': socio-cultural influences on direct observation in medical training. Med Educ 2016;50(10):1054–64.
82. Kogan JR, Hatala R, Hauer KE, et al. Guidelines: the do's, don'ts and don't knows of direct observation of clinical skills in medical education. Perspect Med Educ 2017;6(5):286–305.
83. Lorwald AC, Lahner FM, Greif R, et al. Factors influencing the educational impact of Mini-CEX and DOPS: a qualitative synthesis. Med Teach 2018;40(4):414–20.
84. Young JQ, Sugarman R, Schwartz J, et al. Overcoming the challenges of direct observation and feedback programs: a qualitative exploration of resident and faculty experiences. Teach Learn Med 2020;32(5):541–51.

Moving?

Make sure your subscription moves with you!

To notify us of your new address, find your **Clinics Account Number** (located on your mailing label above your name), and contact customer service at:

Email: journalscustomerservice-usa@elsevier.com

800-654-2452 (subscribers in the U.S. & Canada)
314-447-8871 (subscribers outside of the U.S. & Canada)

Fax number: 314-447-8029

Elsevier Health Sciences Division
Subscription Customer Service
3251 Riverport Lane
Maryland Heights, MO 63043

*To ensure uninterrupted delivery of your subscription,
please notify us at least 4 weeks in advance of move.